Contents

- Introduction
- How it all works
- How to use the scripts
- Relaxation induction 1
- Relaxation induction 2
- Relaxation induction 3
- Relaxation induction 4
- Bringing someone to full waking consciousness
- Confidence and performance anxiety
- Confidence and combatting social anxiety
- Acceptance
- Deep, healing sleep
- Feeling more sure of oneself
- Healing river
- Removing health anxiety/conflict resolution/inner peace
- Overcoming pain
- Withstanding fear
- Coping with illness, increasing well being
- Finding meaning in life
- Creating resilience
- Final note

Do not wait for leaders; do it alone, person to person.
Mother Teresa

During my long career as a psychotherapist I've been privileged to work with a large number of people from all backgrounds, ethnicities, ages; people bringing problems and emotional distresses I never could have imagined when I first started practising over thirty years ago. It has been my intention to help every single person using the best of my knowledge and ability.

Back then I'd trained in hypnotherapy to complement my practice, as well as numerous other therapeutic approaches, and I found my practice was going very well, with lots of recommendations and satisfied clients.

I soon realised the helpfulness of using relaxation and hypnotherapy within the therapy hour. I noticed how much more calm and reassured clients felt after just twenty minutes of 'hypno'-therapeutic relaxation regardless of the issues they brought with them to my therapy room. I've been using the techniques and method ever since.

It is important to understand that hypnosis or guided imagery is an easy thing to learn and do. When you read the chapter on how brain waves affect levels of activity in our brains you'll appreciate how hypnosis is something happening to all of us every day and is a natural part of our daily experiences. We just don't really notice it.

Being trained in NLP, a form of therapy using language as a means to create positive change, I began using more creative verbal statements with clients during hypnotherapy sessions to better help them feel better. By using emphasis on certain words, such as '**feel better**' and changing the tone and pace of my talking voice I was aware the subconscious mind focusses in on those words or phrases and takes notice of them in particular. In this way the subconscious mind can put together another meaning in addition to the surface layer that is being said.

Here's an example;

"**I'm** *thinking the clock on the wall is working* **much better** *now that it's equipped* **with** *new batteries for* **more energy**."

If you piece together the words emphasised in **bold** you'll notice they make another sentence,

"I'm much better with more energy."

The subconscious mind hears this sentence even though the conscious mind is likely to not hear it. This is because the conscious mind is focussed on listening to the whole sentence about the clock, on processing the message in the sentence, deciding whether or not to accept it, criticise it, categorise it, or any number of other things the conscious mind can do. The subconscious mind quietly and without judgement, accepts the message absolutely, sending responses throughout the body if necessary and within the brain. It is instrumental in changing the types and levels of chemicals being released into the body. In summary, all of this is a good thing.

I devised many helpful phrases I could use and remember, which I slipped into sentences as clients enjoyed a relaxing guided visualisation or hypnotherapy as part of their therapeutic journey. I felt heart warmed to receive reports back from client after client saying that they'd been transformed through this method, and I noted this type of therapy was a quicker approach than many others.

I began to think about how else I could help more people. Thinking about it was the start of the book you're reading right now. I realised the relaxation method is not hard to do - anyone can put emphasis on certain useful words, but what is difficult is knowing what to say and remembering what, how and when to say it. So I wrote out relaxation inductions, some of which are complied together in this book. You can use them. You don't have to be able to put someone in an hypnotic trance to use them, you just have to encourage them to become as relaxed as possible. To do that I've written four initial simple relaxation scripts which are at the beginning of the book that you can choose from, and then use these with one of the inductions you've chosen for a particular purpose.

It really is as simple as that. You need a genuine and willing person whom for whatever reasons could benefit from one or more of the scripts here, prepare your calm and quiet space, then begin to speak.
Speak slowly with one tone of voice except when putting emphasis on the phrases in bold, then say those words with more emphasis.

You can find some demonstrations of me using the scripts on youtube. Search for my name, hypnotherapy induction scripts, and demonstration and you'll find them.
I think this approach will be of benefit to **most people** without reservation because the subconscious mind **will** ignore anything that it **find**s isn't useful or **helpful** to the person so you can make the **suggestions** feeling confident **that** you will be **mak**ing **a** positive **difference** to someone **for the better**!

How does it work?

If you're confident in speaking the guided imagery inductions in the following chapters you can skip this introduction and start straight away. This chapter simply gives a background explanation of how you can change the brain into a relaxed state, how it's simple to use once you know how, and it's completely natural, which can be reassuring to know.

Firstly, let's find out what brain relaxation is and how it's a form of hypnotherapy:
It's just a natural part of brainwave activity; it's simply something we can tap in to, something that can help us feel better.
Relaxation and hypnotherapy are very closely related, being part of the family of differing frequencies of brainwave activity. Brainwaves are coordinated electrical 'beats' coming from huge numbers of neuronal interactions. These beats or pulses happen extremely rapidly and are measured in Hertz. One hertz is one cycle per second.
There are five names for differing speeds of brainwaves:
Gamma
Beta
Alpha
Theta
Delta

Gamma waves: around 40 hertz - 100 hertz This is the brainwave speed where we learn the most, we think and preform well. However, too much for too long causes anxiety, too little causes depression. Meditation increases gamma wave activity in our brains. Gamma waves are often present in the four other waves below. They don't tend to 'stand alone'.

Beta waves: around 12 hertz - 40 hertz This is the speed of brainwave activity where we're alert, we can focus on activities and thoughts. Our memory is clearest and we can problem solve. If we have too much beta for too long we will feel stressed and anxious. If we have too little we tend to daydream or feel depressed. Coffee and other stimulants increase beta waves.

Alpha waves: around 8 hertz - 12 hertz This speed is good for light relaxation. If we have too much for too long we will feel dreamy and unable to focus. If we have too little we'll feel anxious, be unable to sleep. We may experience OCD. To increase alpha waves there is alcohol, certain antidepressants and other relaxing substances.

Theta waves: around 4 - 8 hertz Using these brainwave speeds we are creative, deeply relaxed. we feel emotional closeness to others and have a sense of intuition. Too little and too long in this range causes stress and deficient emotional acuity. Too much and we feel depressed, impulsive and sometimes hyperactive. To increase theta waves we can use depressants.

Delta waves: around 0 - 4 hertz These speeds are good for the immune system and creating natural physical healing. In delta wave we enjoy deep restorative sleep. Too much delta waves and we encounter problems learning and thinking. Not enough delta waves causes inadequate sleep, inability to wake up properly and inability to rejuvenate. To increase delta waves we must sleep more, or use depressants.

To enjoy the beneficial effects of deep relaxation, or hypnotherapy, the best brainwave speeds to be in are alpha, theta and delta. This means the body and the mind must be slowed and calmed before healing and changes take place in those three lower brainwave speeds. Much useful beneficial therapy takes place in theta wavebands.
It makes sense then, to slow the brain waves down, to become calmer and more relaxed in our thinking, feelings and thoughts. This book can help you do that.

So, now we know about slowing down our brainwaves, how do we use the scripts in this book? Turn to the next chapter....

How to use the Scripts.

Almost everyone who can speak can use this book to help others, by talking to them. Sounds simple? It's almost as simple as that. There are a few changes you'll have to make to your usual speaking voice which are easy to do once you've practised a bit. Whilst speaking out loud for thirty minutes to someone who isn't going to reply might seem daunting at first, I promise you you'll get used to it. The more you talk the easier it becomes. Remember that your aim is to be useful and effective in helping someone to feel better, as this can spur you on to ignore any embarrassment you may feel or uncertainty about if you're doing it right or not. You can't really do it wrong, that's the great thing about these guided imageries. You are reading a script, it's the listener's subconscious mind that does the main thing, which is to create images and thoughts for the listener to imagine and enjoy as you speak.

There are examples of myself speaking guided imageries on youtube. You may wish to listen to these before you try yourself. See the last chapter of this book for more information on how to find these.

Speak slowly and calmly as you read the script. Use a lower tone. Avoid high pitches, or any higher sounds. Keep the sound of your voice as natural yet as low as you can. You may wish to play background music. Softer, relaxing music is better for helping the brain to relax.

There are three dots (…) after a comma throughout each script to indicate when to stop speaking. Each dot represents about one second, but you can be flexible with the pauses depending on how relaxed your subject is. Generally the more relaxed the person is the longer you can maintain pauses.

In some places the scripts have five dots after the comma (.....) At these places make a slightly longer pause.

The pauses give the brain time to process information and allows relaxation to embed.
Look at your subject often as you speak. Ensure they are relaxed and becoming more relaxed. If they look tense or alert spend more time talking them through the physical relaxation which is used at the beginning of every induction.

Embedded sentences:
Some of the words are highlighted in **bold.** Make a stress on these words, such as more of an emphasis, slightly louder, or draw out the word longer than the others. This is to give a signal to the subconscious mind that the words is somehow different than the others. The words in bold, when seen together, make other sentences that the conscious mind will not pick up on but the subconscious mind will. In this way the mind receives those embedded sentences as facts or 'commands' which are true. The mind starts to make them true by changing thought processes and perceptions. This is one of the basic tenets of hypnotherapy guided imagery.

To help someone become more alert at the end of an induction:
As the script comes to an end you can begin to talk at a gentle but more normal pace. If you're playing music in the background be

ready to turn it off when you want the person to open their eyes and 'come back to the room'. Some of the inductions allow for a person to float off into a healing sleep where you wouldn't bring them back to awareness. The inductions that ask a person to wake up can be ended by slowly counting from 3 to 1, telling the person that they will open their eyes on the count of 1, feeling rested, alert and focussed.

Be prepared to talk through the inductions a few times as a practice before using on someone else. Get used to saying the sentences out loud and stressing the words in bold.
You can do this, and I wish you every success.

To make things a little more simple, think of the process as three steps:

1. **Prepare.** Make yourself and the listener/s as comfortable as possible, in a quiet where you're unlikely to be interrupted. Coach your listener by explaining you're going to be talking for around thirty minutes.
2. **Deliver**. Have a glass of water on hand for yourself. Then begin to talk, checking your speed is slow enough and your tone and volume is suitable.
3. **Finish well.** After you've finished spend some moments talking with your listener about everyday things, if possible asking them simple questions about the rest of their day. Allow them to sleep if it's OK for them to do so.

The next five chapters consist of four standard initial relaxation scripts which you can use before starting your chosen induction to help your subject (friend, family member, or other) begin to relax

deeper, and one ending paragraph of a chapter. The ending one is to help your subject to awaken from the guided imagined journey you've taken them on. Simply decide which of the first initial ones you'd like to use or follow the suggestion at the beginning of each chapter for which to use. Then at the end of the induction if you wish to use the standard awakening script you just speak it after completing the full guided imagery script or induction.
(This should make more sense to you once you begin to use the scripts.)

The final two inductions are longer in length, and offer the opportunity to try out slightly more complex use of language and linguistics to create positive change. There's nothing special you have to do, keep using your voice the same as with the others, and following the instructions above.

All of the inductions use metaphor as a helpful tool for change, and the last two inductions are no exception. The use of contrast or dual meanings are also beneficial in encouraging the subconscious mind to accept what is being said. The use of absolute contrast of two opposing elements, such as night time and daytime is another method to help someone stay relaxed and receptive to what is being said to them. Give them a try!

Physical relaxation induction number 1.

Say the words slowly, in rhythm with a calm steady tone. This induction should take around five to ten minutes.

Find a comfortable position,…
Free from disturbance,…
For around half an hour,…
Your clothing is loose,…
And you're pleasantly warm,…
Any noises are unimportant,…
Let yourself begin to relax,…
Focussing on your feet,…
which are warm and comfortable,…
Feel your feet relaxing more,…
That feeling spreads into your ankles,…
Then your shins and calves,…
So soft and loose,…
Letting go of muscle tension,…
Breathing easily and naturally,…
The relaxation continues to your upper thighs,…
Where you're beginning to feel heavier,…
In a good way,…
So soft and warm,…
Then your hips are more relaxed,…
And your waist,…
Your stomach releases unwanted tension,…
As you feel yourself drifting pleasantly,…
Into a state of comfort,…
And a sense of wellbeing,…
As your back lets go of muscle tension,…
Just let it happen,…
Just notice your chest becoming softer,…
With a sense of relief,…
A good feeling,…
Now focus on your shoulders relaxing,…
your neck,…
And your upper arms, elbows and lower arms,…
Hands, fingers and thumbs,…
All relaxed,…
Continuing to breath easily and naturally,…
Letting go of unwanted negative thoughts,…

Along with unwanted feelings,…
Should they return,…
Simply notice them,…
Then allow them to drift away,…
without judgement,…
As your head rests heavily on the surface beneath it,…
The muscles of your face are still,…
So much more relaxed,…
And the whole of your body feels heavy,…
Sinking into the surface beneath it,…
Whilst at the same time,…
You're feeling lighter than air,…
And sometimes,…
You won't be aware of your body,…
Just the sound of my voice,…
That will help you,…
From now on,…
Let that happen,…
Right now,…

Induction for standard physical relaxation number 2.

This is a longer version than number 1. It should take between 10 and 15 minutes to talk through this one. Use this induction rather than induction 1 if your subject appears very physically tense. Speak more slowly than usual, and use a soft and low tone of voice.

Make yourself comfortable, prepare yourself to relax as much as it is possible right now,…sitting or laying down in the best place for you, …right now,…so you can relax more and more,…drifting off to a place of absolute comfort of your physical self,…where as much as you can,…you can find relief in letting go of unwanted tensions,… throughout your body,…just by using the power of your mind to focus on different parts of your body,…enabling them to become so much more soft and warm,…gently encouraging the muscles to become softer,…whereby you're able to let go absolutely,…which is the way you begin to feel so much better,……
So right now,…take the focus of your attention to the soles of your feet and the muscles within the soles of your feet,…allowing those muscles to rest and relax,…feeling the warm glow emanating from them as you do that,…because you're focussing on the souls of your feet all other noises are unimportant to you,…you are unaware of them,…as that soft, warm feeling spreads to the whole of your feet, … as you let the whole of your feel become loose and limp and very comfortable,…keep focussing on how relaxed your feet are,…as you take a large breath in, filling your lungs,…then breath out very slowly, …embracing the relief your body feels as you let go of the breath,… and once more breathing in a full lungs' breath,…and breathing out very slowly,…now move the focus of your attention to your ankles,… and your mind lets your ankle muscles relax,…and your calf muscles, your shins,…becoming softer, warmer, much more pleasant,…because as you relax in this way,…so your body can

begin to recover,…and let go of all the unnecessary and unwanted tensions within your physical self,…so that you can begin to relax totally,…in every way,……

and that feeling of relaxation spreads to your upper thighs,…as the sensation of relaxation moves like a wave of loving energy,…travelling up your body,…calming,…soothing,…relaxing,…as you allow that to happen,…so you will begin to feel so much better,…simply listen to the sound of my voice,…as your subconscious mind follows the instructions to relax,….you will sink into a state of wellbeing where you are comforted,…where you are safe,…and things feel much better,…because continuing to relax in this way, physically, using your natural breath to help relaxation,…is the best approach to letting go,…and preparing to drift off into a wonderful place of comfort, harmony and peaceful serenity,…so that your body welcomes the sensations which reassure, comfort with a care that is soft yet powerful,…then you can focus your attention on your hips, allowing them to feel the wave of loving, healing, soothing energy caress and soften,…as the feeling of letting go and stillness moves to your waist and stomach,…let your stomach muscles let go,…and your back,…so that you can sink into the surface beneath you,…deeper and deeper,…enjoying the flow of energy,…as your chest relaxes,…your clavicle and your shoulders,…all softer,…breathing rhythmically and naturally,…your upper arms have let go,…your elbows, lower arms, wrists,…your hands, fingers and thumbs,…realising it is so healthy to do this,…to relax your body so completely, …as much as you can,…as your neck muscles just let go,…so your head feels heavier,…it relaxes, as the wave of energy reaches the crown of your head and the muscles beneath the crown of your head relax,…your scalp muscles are relaxing,…feel the muscles under the skin of your forehead relax,…as if someone is kindly and gently stroking your forehead,…and the muscles around your eyes are relaxing,…behind your eyes,…relaxing,…as the muscles of your cheeks feel full, warm,…soft,…just as the muscles around your lips soften,…your lips feel full, warm and still,…and your jaw is loose,…your tongue is loose inside your mouth,…so that right now,…you feel completely dreamy,…your body is feeling very heavy,…yet at the same time it feels as light as air,…as if you could float around the room,…even at times, you are not aware of your body at all,……

Relaxation induction number 3. (non physical)

This relaxation introduction will take around five to ten minutes. Follow the flow of the words, resting for a few seconds when you come to the comma and full stops.

Take a deep breath, filling your lungs then holding the breath for the count of five,…one,…two,…three,…four,…five,…that's it, good,…now breathe out slowly and steadily,…as slowly as you can,…then take in another full breath holding it for the count of five once more, …one,…two,…three,…four,…five,…and now continue to breathe naturally and easily without thinking about it,…at all,…being subconsciously aware that when you breathe in you're breathing in clean fresh air,…that will energise you,…helping to cleanse and strengthen you,…and with every out breath you make you're removing unwanted waste products from your body and lungs, getting rid of toxins that are no longer necessary,…so you will maintain a healthy rhythm of in breaths and out breaths as you allow yourself to feel the relaxation which comes along with breathing in,…and breathing out,…that is perfect healthy and exactly the way it is all the time,…so you feel a deeper sense of being calm and peaceful,…which increases as you allow that to happen, and enjoy the feelings of letting go,…imagine you are floating upwards towards the ceiling,…you are lighter than air, enjoying this experience,…where you are in control with a sense of curiosity as you float higher and higher,…so that as you reach the ceiling you find you're able to float straight through it,…upwards, higher and higher,…feeling safe and secure,…looking around you as you glide upwards,…you've travelled through the top of the building and are floating in the sky,…

where you move your body this way and that way,…because you have full control of your movements and find that you can direct where you go to by moving, tilting in the direction you're aiming for,…then you can look down and see all the house below you looking so small,…the roads, cars, gardens,…in fact everything you see below you is so far away the view resembles a model town where everything seems unreal,…and that's fine,…because sometimes it's helpful to take another perspective like this,…where the importance of somethings diminish,…seem so far away,…as you float in another direction, towards the sea,…where the smell in the air becomes filled with the aromas of seaweeds, salty sea water,…and seagulls fly past you,…they are friendly and happy to see you there,…all the while you're breathing in,…and out,…in,…and out,…looking at ships sailing the middle of the ocean,…wind farms,…gliding, floating calmly along,…understanding that you have the power to return to the place where you began your journey when ever you wish,…because you're in control,…with the ability to direct where you go,…even as you are so very relaxed and comfortable,…just as you can imagine floating lighter than air in the sky,…so you can imagine making the changes to your thoughts and feelings,…without having to think about it right now,…just let it happen,…and it will happen,…because in relaxing so much you will find the right directions for yourself,…allowing you subconscious mind to take you to where you wish to be,…from now on,…as you float back through the sky to the building where you began your journey,…back though the ceiling,…back to the room,..to where you were resting,…you're there again now,…breathing in and out,…in and out,…feeling so much more at ease,…ready to continue, listening to the sound of my voice,…as you let it happen,…

Induction for relaxation number 4. (non physical)

This initial relaxation should take about five to ten minutes. Use this induction with someone who is already fairly relaxed. Speak softly and slowly, taking rests where you see the comma and three dots.

There are many ways to relax yourself,…you can get lots of sleep which is good for you in every way,…perhaps you enjoy lighthearted films that lift your spirits,…I wonder what your favourite films are,…and I wonder if you've watched one of them recently,…because if you have then you're already relaxed simply be thinking about that film and remembering how happy you felt,…as you can notice how you are becoming more and more relaxed here and now as you listen to my voice encouraging you to let go and relax more and more,…feeling a gentle calm confidence in knowing you are going to feel so much better after listening to the whole of the messages and suggestions the sound of my voice brings to you to help you,…in every way you wish for,……

realising there are indeed many many other ways to relax yourself without having to even try, just by remembering relaxing times you've had in the past,…those comforting and comfortable feelings of being present in the moment remembering the time when the moment was lovely,…just what you needed,…bringing it to the present time,…feeling those feelings all over again,…or you can relax as you imagine a beautiful scene or image in your mind's eye,…maybe a countryside rich in greens of flora and fauna,…or a seaside beach image where it's as if you can smell the fresh salty sea air,…as well as the song of seagulls flying in the sky above,…as you lay on the soft white sand which is warm from the heat of the sun above,…all this can relax you,…taking your focus of attention to healthier thoughts and to better feelings,…so you can begin a journey into deeper and deeper relaxation without you having to do anything else other than let it happen,……

because as you let go more and more,…so your subconscious mind will take the reins and guide you towards all you wish to achieve for yourself inwardly,…giving you strength and resolve where its needed,…encouraging and taking action to help you begin to achieve your aims,…listening to only those suggestions that will help you,…whilst allowing your conscious mind to listen without judgement,…accepting that the subconscious mind is most wise,…most caring and considerate of what is good for you,…from now on, …so just allow this to happen,…whether you're thinking about the lighthearted film you recently watched,…or whether you're remembering a time in the past when you were very relaxed,…or you're imagining you're in the countryside,…or at a beautiful beach, …or even at the top of a mountain, surrounded by mountain ranges on all sides,…you can enjoy this sensation of becoming more and more, deeper and deeper relaxed,…

Bringing someone to full waking consciousness
(after having completed the chosen induction)

*This is a general script that can be used with all the guided imagery inductions to bring a person to
a state of being alert.*

….. ….. ….. …..

…so,…as you feel how very relaxed you are,…so relaxed that it can feel as if you are fast asleep,…in fact you are in a state of pre-sleep, …where you are not asleep,…and you are not fully awake,…which is a very lovely place to be,…as your body is able to heal much more easily in this state,…as well as you being able to let your thoughts drift away,…to allow your subconscious mind to find solutions for you,…to any questions you may have,…without you having to even think about them,…you will find that in a few moments,…when you wake up fully,…you will have a much better idea of what the answers to those questions could be,…all the while staying absolutely calm, …rested,…filled with relief,…with a strong sense of well being throughout your body,…because you'll feel as if you've been asleep, …even though you haven't,…..

now,…very slowly,…take steady breaths and keeping steady thoughts,…I'm going to count from 3 to 1 to begin to bring you back to full waking consciousness,…in the gentlest possible way,…so right now I'm counting number **3**,…and you're beginning to be aware of the sound of my voice being much nearer to you,…and you're becoming aware of other sounds that may be in the room, or even outside of the room,…just notice these sounds,…as I count number **2**,…and with your eyelids still closed, your body still and relaxed,… you're beginning to remember the colour scheme in the room,…and the position of the furniture here in this room, right now,…and you are getting a sense of where you are in relation to the different pieces of furniture,…and you're ready now to think about opening your eyes as I count number **1**,…because you can,…whenever you're ready,…open your eyes,…slowly if you like,…and start to focus on something ahead of you,…maybe a picture on the wall,…or another object,…that's good,…take a couple of deeper breaths,… yes, that's it,…have a full stretch of your body,…like a cat does,… that's really good,…well done you,…and welcome back,…

Confidence and Performance Anxiety

no preliminary induction is needed for this script

Alright now,…as you allow yourself to clear your mind of all thoughts you've brought with you,…letting them float away from you,…so your mind can rest,…and your subconscious mind is moved to the foreground of your thinking,…so you can allow your body to rest and relax,…finding the peace and calm that will help you drift into a wonderful state of transformation,…where your conscious mind can choose to listen to the sound of my voice,…and to the words and suggestions that will help you to be, and feel, and act in the ways that you wish for,…or your conscious mind can choose not to listen, that's absolutely fine,…because your conscious mind can allow thoughts to drift in and out as I continue to speak,…bringing helpful messages and suggestions that will be heard by your subconscious mind,…so that your subconscious mind will take notice of all the messages,…of all helpful, useful, sensible suggestions that help change for the better,…for you,…and then implement those changes for you,…because your subconscious mind, whilst usually quiet and subdued on the surface, is actually the most important part of your mind,…and is deep deep deep and wide,…and it's the subconscious mind's role to order and guide everything you do in life,…so simply rest and relax,…being sure that you don't have to do anything at all other than allow yourself to drift and float,…becoming more and more comfortable,…feeling the muscles of your body softening,…feeling the warmth of your body,…and just letting your body become loose and limp,…at ease,…and from now on each time I use the word now,…just like that, 'now',…you will sink deeper and deeper into that subconscious state,..of peace and harmony,…where change will take place for the better,…from now on,…so feeling the weight of your head as it rests against the surface beneath **you**,… also feeling the warmth throughout your body,…as you **perform** this act of relaxing,…and just noticing places in your body that maybe you can **well** sense movement,…or tightness,…focus on those places one at once and then let it go,…and in and **under** your mind's eye visualise yourself, without any **pressure**,…sitting at the bottom of a green hill,…and you're looking up at the grass and the wild flowers and the sky above,…because the grass and wild flowers, some trees and bushes are growing up the hillside,…and be aware of the warm breeze blowing gently on your cheeks and through your hair,…and enjoying the fresh smells of the countryside as you sit in the valley,…looking upwards,…feeling the sun warming **you**,…and as you sit there,…you **are** reflective,…and the amazing fact that your body is made of atoms,…billions upon billions of atoms,…**confident**, tiny movements of energy resonating at and **in** different levels and speeds,…creating you,…an **all** thinking, feeling, acting human,…and realising that the surface beneath you is also made of atoms,… **situations** of moving energy,…and we can move your energy within your body to create absolute success for you,…where what needs to change changes,…and you become contented,…satisfied,…and happy because your subconscious mind has the power to do that,… and within one atom there is so much space,…so much more space, …with protons neutrons, electrons,…so much space,…between them,…comparatively,…so **you are** amazing,…miraculous,…and you can be filled with awe and wonder,…and **stronger** in your mind's eye you stand **and** breathe in steadily and well,…deep into your lungs at a **stronger** pace,…then you begin to climb up the hillside,…and I wonder whether **emotionally** you will choose to climb straight up the hillside to get there quicker,…or whether you will walk more gently round and round the hill,…or even maybe you will fly to the top of the hillside,…because you can do that using the power of your visualisation in your mind,…however you do that you're now standing at the top of the hillside looking beyond the hill at an enormous mountain behind it,…and it would be a challenge for you to climb this mountain,…and you feel compelled to find out how far you can go,…**so** maybe you will climb to the top,…or maybe you will climb halfway,…then being **sure**, you decide to make that journey,…to do that as a challenge to yourself,…and feeling very confident with absolutely trust **of yourself**,…you begin to make the journey upwards,…and you look to the left and you look to the right as you're climbing,…constantly looking all around for places to hold on to for places to put your feet securely,… and with that natural tenacity of yours where your intrepid spirit guides you,…surefooted and with poise,…showing courage and mettle,…you begin to feel the satisfaction of starting that journey upwards,…you're calm,…even though what you're doing is daring,…you're **happy** and decisive,…because you have absolute belief in yourself and your ability,…its a potent, mighty feeling **to be** making your way up this enormous rock face of a mountain,…and **in** such positiveness,…feeling secure and together,…using your **full** resourcefulness,…and your cleverness,…you're now standing at the top of the mountain,…with an amazing **view**,…and in your minds eye look all around you,…behind you there is a huge building made **of** stone, grey stone, it could be a monastery or a large school or some workplace for **people**,…everything is quiet and still,…the air is thinner,…and you can see for miles and miles in all directions,…and as you stand there your feet apart, strong, sturdy,…calm full of self-reliance,…a life force comes into **you** and you accept and **enjoy** all those qualities that have been proven by your journey to the top of this mountain,…you're better at **talking**,…you have absolute self assurance of your innate ability **to** succeed,…and with this life force you've gained stamina,…an essence within you which is substantial to yourself and to **others**,… now enter the building,…because you're curious about this building as a place or refuge,…a place of life,…vibrancy, dynamism,… newness, and as you walk past the hallway you enter a large hall full of people,…all looking at **you** as you take a deep breath of surprise, …because you **have** seen there is stage at the end of the hall, and the audience are sitting, waiting for you to stand on that stage,…and **increasing** your courage,…and your strength,…your **confidence,** and your clear headed sense of power,…without having to think ab**out** it,…as you stand on that stage,….you find you're **going** to talk easily, comfortably, naturally,…saying interesting things,…pertinent, …you have so much to say,…the audience is enraptured by your words and **characteristics**,…there's a pizzaz to your delivery,…and as one or more of the audience ask questions so you can talk more **naturally**, and more,…and more, and you're feeling within yourself such a sense of verve and bounce,…like you're gaining energy from speaking,…and you're enjoying being listened to,…you feel a keenness within you to deliver the messages that come to you in your head,…and you're well aware that you have a real presence on that stage,…and that the audience is eager to hear more from you,… they're spellbound by your words, receptive to everything you say,… importantly you're feeling animated,…and delighted,…eventually everybody is applauding you,…they're cheering and whistling and smiling and somebody in the wings of the stage motions for you to follow them,…and you follow them backstage through corridors,… and then to a door,…and you enter the room by yourself and there are three people sitting at a desk smiling and you sit opposite,…and even though these are new people to you they're asking you all sorts of questions about yourself that you love to answer,…and you can feel there interest in you,…and you can appreciate,…how much you can say and how useful you can be,…and with every word you utter **you're feeling so good** about yourself,…you have a push and a drive to say more and to show them,…how proficient **you are**,…and how resourceful and **masterly** you have been in your life and can be **from now on**,…and the room swells with an atmosphere of understanding,…of acceptance,…harmony and serenity,…and you're feeling so well and healthy this shines out from you,…and these three people smile and thank you for answering their questions,…and helping them,…and so you stand and leave the room,…where a kindly person leads you further down corridors in this huge stone building,…until you reach a bedroom,…and as you enter the bedroom you can see an enormous four poster bed in the centre of the room with the bedposts against the wall,…and the view from the window is idyllic and again you take deep breaths of pride and satisfaction at your achievements,…and at your performance,… and you feel stronger, taller,…relaxed,…giving yourself absolute credit,…for being yourself,…up and then you take yourself to the bed and rest your body on the sumptuous mattress,…your head lays on the sunken pillow,…and you allow yourself to fall into a deep loving, soothing, healing sleep,…and you sleep deeper and deeper,…a sleep, soft gentle loving healing sleep,…sleep of reflection and harmony,…and you sleep so deeply that you begin to dream,…and it's a lovely dream that you welcome,…of transformation for the better,…the dream begins with you sitting at the bottom of a green valley looking up at a green hillside,…sprinkled with wild flowers, and bushes and trees,…and above the sky is blue and the sun is pouring down it's heat and rays upon you,…and you're feeling so good about yourself,…and all is well,…and all will be well,… from now on,…

(If the person wishes to wake up after this induction you can use the longer version of bringing the person to full alertness, found near the beginning of this book and reprinted below):

…so,…as you feel how very relaxed you are,…so relaxed that it can feel as if you are fast asleep,…in fact you are in a state of pre-sleep,…where you are not asleep,…and you are not fully awake,…which is a very lovely place to be,…as your body is able to heal much more easily in this state,…as well as you being able to let your thoughts drift away,…to allow your subconscious mind to find solutions for you,…to any questions you may have,…without you having to even think about them,…you will find that in a few moments,…when you wake up fully,…you will have a much better idea of what the answers to those questions could be,…all the while staying absolutely calm,…rested,…filled with relief,…with a strong sense of well being throughout your body,…because you'll feel as if you've been asleep,…even though you haven't,……

*now,…very slowly,…take steady breaths and keeping steady thoughts,…I'm going to count from 3 to 1 to begin to bring you back to full waking consciousness,…in the gentlest possible way,…so right now I'm counting number **3**,…and you're beginning to be aware of the sound of my voice being much nearer to you,…and you're becoming aware of other sounds that may be in the room, or even outside of the room,…just notice these sounds,…as I count number **2**,…and with your eyelids still closed, your body still and relaxed,…you're beginning to remember the colour scheme in the room,…and the position of the furniture here in this room, right now,…and you are getting a sense of where you are in relation to the different pieces of furniture,…and you're ready now to think about opening your eyes as I count number **1**,…because you can,…whenever you're ready,…open your eyes,…slowly if you like,…and start to focus on something ahead of you,…maybe a picture on the wall,…or another object,…that's good,…take a couple of deeper breaths,…yes, that's it,…have a full stretch of your body,…like a cat does,…that's really good,…well done you,…and welcome back,…*

Increase Confidence and Combat Social Anxiety

No standard induction is necessary.

First of all, take in a deep breath, fill your lungs and hold that breath,…one, two, three, four, five,…then very slowly breathe out and let go of unwanted tension as you do so,…that's good,…and now another deep breath in,…hold it for,…two, three, four, five, and then a very slow breath out,…as you rest and relax your physical body,…feeling your muscles becoming loose and limp as you do so,…rested,…simply letting go,…more and more,…another deep breathe in and then continue breathing naturally,…and in your usual style,…and we're going to begin by relaxing your physical body first,…then we will focus on helping your emotions to change to become more positive and uplifting,…as you let go of unwanted physical and emotional feelings,…letting go of all those that are no longer necessary,…or are unhelpful,…and then we will enable your subconscious mind to process your ways of thinking and feeling,…so that your behaviour and your ways of thinking will change for the better from now on,…in the ways that you wish to for the better,…helping you to become so much more your true real self,…where ***you*** can ***feel*** fulfilled,…***satisfied and enriched*** in your daily life,…and continuing that natural easy breathing,…***being aware*** that with each breath you breathe out you're breathing out the unwanted waste products of breath,…the toxins,…and ***each time*** you're breathing in,…***you're*** breathing in clean fresh air that holds oxygen and helpful substances,…***helping*** every single cell of ***your*** body to rest and recover,…heal,…to rejuvenate,…and find full maximum health,...so that the ***whole*** of your body can function with optimum ***performance***,...whilst all the while you're feeling at one with yourself,...***in*** an easy manner,...***feeling good*** about all that you are,...and all your plans and wishes are shaping up,......

and right now,...you can imagine that it is night time,...and the sky outside is dark and ***all is*** still,...and ***peaceful***,...quiet,...and the air is warm,...with a restful atmosphere,...***and*** you're becoming more and more ***comfortable***,...with every breath you breathe in,...and every breath you breathe out,...***so you're*** tranquil,... and ***calm***,...as you take the focus of your attention to the soles of your feet, and the muscles within the soles of your feet,...feeling them with your mind,...feeling the softness as you let go more and more of unwanted tension,...so that your toes become more relaxed,...just as in the same way your upper feet let go,...and rest,...and that feeling of heaviness and peace is spreading into your ankles,...and into ***your*** shins,...softer,...heavier,...just allowing your shins to be at one,...***in harmony***,...your calf muscles,...simply ***allowing*** the natural healing state to come upon ***you***,...so you can rejuvenate,...and ***to recover***,...in all those cells of your body,...***as you*** can sense your knees welcoming this time to ***be calm and still***,...behind your knees,...and your thighs front and back,...your upper thighs feeling the weight of your legs now,...pressing into the surface beneath you as you completely let go,...your hips resting,...healthily and heavily,...***feel*** your hips and notice the ***sensations*** you may have in and around your hips,...your stomach,...and your lower back,...to your waist,...simply in balance,...with a sense ***of feeling right*** in yourself,...as it is,...in the healthiest of ways,...as that sensation of peace,...***of love***,...and harmony spreads in to your stomach,...middle, back, and chest,...and you breathe naturally,...easily,...comfortably,...***while being aware*** of deeper relaxation that is coming upon you,...as you allow yourself to drift into **a wonderful** state of **comfort and safety**, …where all **is working well** for you,…so that your upper back and your shoulders are rested and relaxed and you feel heavier and heavier,…your clavicle and your shoulders,…your upper arms, heavier,…elbows,…lower arms and wrists,…palms of your hands, the backs of your hands,…thumbs **and** fingers,…full,…warm,…soft, so that **you are able,**…to think yourself *in*to this state,…of being so deeply **at one with yourself** and your body,…that the relaxation comforts you and reassures you,…you will be able to continue resting and relaxing,…whilst all you wish for begins to come to fruition,… as your neck and all the muscles within your neck soften so you can feel the weight of your head as it rests upon the surface beneath it… so heavy,…you welcome this feeling of restfulness,… letting go more and more,…as if you're drifting,…allowing yourself to drift,.. encouraging your self,…and you can feel the muscles in your scalp becoming soft,…warm,…and the muscles in your forehead,… softer,…as if some hand loving,…caring,…soothing hand is stroking your forehead,…increasing your sense of safety and wellbeing,…the muscles around your eyes are softer,…and behind your eyes,…so still,…as the muscles in your cheeks feel full and warm,…and your jaw,…is loose as your tongue is loose inside your mouth,…and you can feel the pulsing in your lips as they feel full and soft,…and you continue to physically rest and relax,…as your subconscious mind and your conscious mind listens to the sound of my voice,…with the messages and suggestions the sound of my voice brings to you,… and whilst your conscious mind can choose to listen to the messages and suggestions that will help you,…from now on,…that the sound of my voice brings,…your conscious mind can choose not to listen to all those messages,…because your subconscious mind will continue listening to everything that is helpful to you,…that the sound of my voice brings,…whilst your subconscious mind will also begin the process of change for the better,…for you,…as you drift deeper and deeper into that wonderful state of peace and harmony, …your subconscious mind is beginning to **enable** the whole of yourself to start **a new process of well being**,…**and** change and **positive thinking**,…of recovery,…so you will gain much more of all those things you wish for,…from this moment on,…and each time you hear me use the word now,… just like that,…now,…so you will become more and more relaxed,…letting go more and more of residual tensions within your body,…so you are **increasingly feeling** light and **happy**,…as you drift in your mind,…to a beautiful place that you can see right now in your mind's eye,…where it is daytime and you're in the countryside,…the sun is shining high in the sky,…ahead of you **you** can see fields upon fields of corn,…wheat,…barley,… maize,…beautiful fields,…beyond which **are** undulating hills,…and to the left of you you can see larger green hills,…**so** far in the distance there are trees on the tops of the hills,…looking so small yet **sure** from where you are,…and to the right **of** you is a dense thick, vibrant forest,…with green leaves,…and brown bark on the trunks,…lush and inviting,…of **yourself**,…it feels friendly,…and you're walk**in**g along a dusty path,…with **all** the time you need,…enjoying the heat of the sun on your face,…through your hair,…through your clothes, …as **you** amble happily along,…breathing in the fresh country smells as you **do** that,…noticing from time to time, wild flowers growing at the side of the path,…and feeling reconnected with your inner,…deep,…carefree self,…that sense of freedom of simply being at one with all parts of you,…whilst at the same time being connected intrinsically to the nature all around you,…..

and after some time **you** notice there are two paths leading into the forest,…and I **really** wonder which one you will take for you to

enjoy,…will you take the path on the left to go to the forest, or will you take the path on the right to go to the forest,…***being*** such a thoughtful person as you are,…I know whichever you choose is the right choice for you,…and ***with*** decisiveness you're now walking on that path,…not any of the ***others***,…you're entering the forest where the atmosphere changes,…it becomes more humid,…***and*** dense,…its colder and darker,…you like that sense of closeness in the forest, …its a good feeling for you,…as if the forest is ***talking*** to you,…and ***with*** the rich forest smells your feelings of well being and ***connectedness*** to yourself are enhanced,…so with a steady pace you begin to walk along the path,…hearing twigs crack beneath your feet as you walk on the moss,…and ***you*** can see slight movements of woodland animals,…between the trunks of the trees,…and you ***have*** the smell the bark in your nostrils,…and above ***lots of*** leaves are rustling in the slight warm breeze,…creating a canopy above you,…and you feel so completely safe, with new-found ***confidence***…as if the forest welcomes you ***and*** cares for you,…and ***you can*** hear the sound of birds high above in the branches, ***express***ing themselves with their different calls,…the sparrows,… robins,…jays,…and blackbirds,…some blue tits,…and because this is your forest created by you for ***yourself***,…there are parrots,… toucans,… peacocks,…cockatoos,……

all at once day turns to night,…and its dark ***in*** the forest,…you can hear the owls,…hooting with ***social*** calls to the wild,…welcoming new ***situations*** to discover,…and when you look up through the leaves on the trees,…you can see the stars in the dark blue night sky,…where the moon is shining down,…as you continue ambling contentedly,…and the trees become larger,…***you're*** entering an ancient part of the forest,…where the trees have lived strong and ***true*** for hundreds and hundreds of years,…and as you stand alone, by your**self**, you can see their trunks are huge,…and their roots gnarled and twisted,…as it **is** clear they have grown down deep into the ground below,…and you notice that on one particularly large and **strong** tree there seems to be light shining from below,…a **confident** glow,…underneath one of the roots,…which is a root that is wider and larger than yourself,…**and** when you look down underneath the root,…you can see several **steady** steps leading down to something underground **which is** lit by light down there,…now you decide thats it's **wise** to make that journey underneath the root and ground,…and you can count ten steps down to that underground place,…and with each step down you're falling deeper and deeper to that wonderful state of well being and contentedness,…deeper and deeper,…one,…two,…three,…four,…five,…deeper and deeper into a place of healing,…restoration,…comfort,…wellbeing,…positive change,…six,…seven,…eight,…nine,…ten, and you're standing in the most tremendous underground garden that is lit by lanterns in the ceiling in the earth,…a very large room,…and it is amazing,…so, clear your mind,…of all previous thoughts,…when you look at the different plants that grow here which are stunning,…curious,…almost incredible,…beautiful colours rich and deep such as you have never seen before,…**from** huge petals and flowers,…with enticing fragrances rich and delightful,…**now** creating within you a sense of inner power,…**on** to latent energy which is being opened up,…**you'r**e given the means by which to discover,…new ways,…to provide you with power and strength,…and a **sense** of knowledge,…beyond,…all your previous expectations,…and at the end **of** this room you notice there's a small wooden door rounded at the top made of wood panels,…with a large metal ring as a door handle,…you open that door with **confidence**, then step into another room,…which seems to be some sort of study or library,…and there are books from floor to ceiling on each wall and near to one wall a leafy plant **grows** tall,…and again the room is lit by lanterns fastened into the ceiling,…and it's as if by being there you're feeling **more** of the awakening of your inner essence of power **and** energy,…you are soaking up all the knowledge from **all** of the books,…and then you notice someone sitting on the floor,…in the corner,… **is** a young man, …with knees bent and head on his knees,…and you can see that you have **great** ability,…to help,…to encourage and coach the man on the floor,…to stand,…and feel able to take some steps towards you,…because as you look at this man,…you can see he is tentative and unsure,…and without having to think about it you are able to say to him,… the right words,…in the right order,…to reassure him,…he will be well,…and **you** can comfort him and show him the way,…and so after a while,…of you talking with him,…he **smile**s and thanks you and together you go to open the next door,…**at** the other side of the room,…which is made of wood panels,…with a **large** metal ring as a door handle,…**and** when you open this door,…you step into a **larger** room,…**together s**o,… feeling reassured,…more comfortable,…**because** you have been able to help,…one man,… and **this** room has the appearance of a dining room,…and **is** inviting to you,…there are two people sitting at **a** table,…with food in front of them yet they are not eating,…a **sign** they are not happy,…and their hands rest on the table as they look down at their food,…whilst all the while **you can** feel,…how different it is for you to **be so strong** and sure of yourself compared **with** these **people,**…sitting at the table,…and **so** with your companion,…**you** sit next to them and begin to **talk** to them,…saying words that will help them **from now on**,…to feel so much better in every way,…**whilst** you notice as you talk,…you're **feeling good** about being there **with** these **people**,… **because** you are enjoying all being together,…knowing that you're leading the way for these **other people**,…to gain confidence,…strength,…in themselves and in their abilities to communicate,…that **makes you happy**,…so that after some time of talking with these people,…you have have transformed them for the better,…the atmosphere in the room is much lighter,…**more jovial** as the four of you walk towards the other door at the other side of the room,…whilst you notice how eager you are to discover who you will find at the other side of the door,…which is made of wood and is rounded at the top,….and has a circular metal door handle,…therefore when you open this door,…**you are full of**…enjoyment and anticipation,…of who will be in this room and what will you see,…all four of you walk through the door and in this room,…there are ten people of all ages,…all different,…looking at you,…as soon as they see you they smile and you're pleased to see them,…because you have realised how you have so much ability to give direction,…and comfort to others simply by being real,…and appreciating,…how you can be the person,…to give others the sense of strength,…**confidence and well being**,…through your presence **and your innate ability to communicate** on all levels,…accepting this is through your body language,…your facial expressions,…it **means** your spoken language also,…**you are so liked**,…**and** whilst the other thirteen people in this room are different to you in a myriad of ways,…**you're feeling absolutely comfortable** with that fact,…**contented and happy**,…and night time may well have turned to daytime,…and in the corner of this room there are ten steps leading upwards and you can see the light which is daylight above,…and you appreciate,…it is time for all of you to take the steps back to the forest,…and to the countryside and to the land,…..

At this point end the induction by bringing the client back to consciousness or allowing them to continue into sleep proper. If you prefer you can use the standard awakening script near the beginning of the book.

Acceptance

Use standard physical relaxation inductions 2 or 3.

As you become increasingly relaxed,…**notice** how you feel so much more at one with yourself,…and with **your** physical **feelings**,…so that as you notice the rhythm of **your breathing**,…and maybe even of your heartbeat,…whilst your mind **is** feeling much **more** rested,… **calm**,…creating healthier and healthier thoughts which float through your mind like welcome warm breezes,…because as **you** do that,… easily and naturally,…only **accept**able, comfortable **feelings** float in and out of your mind,…bringing for you relief,…a letting go,…of unwanted energies,…which are unnecessary in your life,…so that as they diminish and leave your thought processes,….you can **allow yourself** to appreciate the sense of **freedom** you feel,…which is accompanied by rising joy,…as well as huge amounts of hopefulness **and** increasing **wellbeing**,…knowing that as this happens to **you**, right now,…your ability to use your imagination increases,…so much more,…which in turn means you're relaxing much more,…**creat**ing slower brain waves,…which are helpful to your sense of **peace** and harmony,…whereby your visual skills become keen,…helping you to **accept** absolutely brilliant images in your mind's eye,…wherein right at this moment,…imagine, right **now**, that you're enjoying a gentle, slow walk through fields,…where you're surrounded by green and beautiful lush countryside,…all the while **you can** smell fresh, clear air,…with each step you take,…bringing with it fragrances of trees,… grass,…flowers,…as well as a pleasant cleansing aroma from the river that is flowing happily on its way to the sea,…far far in the distance,…now, as **you accept** the long meandering, winding route this river takes,…as a way of being at one with all nature surrounding you,…you focus on **how** the river **is** twisting and turning,…making graceful movements towards the destination of the stunning golden seashore,…some way in the distance,…even though you can not see that far ahead,…you realise **what will transpire** with each step you take,… **is** that you're becoming so very relaxed,…increasingly relaxed,…falling deeper and deeper into a place of **absolute** harmony,…of contentment,…a **comfortable,** welcome sensation where all unwanted ideas and thoughts have disappeared,…for good,…because when that happens you relax even more,…becoming interested to **notice** how they have no interest to you at all,…as if they never had any effect upon you,…in the first place,…in fact instead, you're filled with **wonderful joy**,… exhilaration at the freeing effect of being so relieved,…and being totally without negative thinking or feelings in any way,…after all,… **you are** so very **capable** and recognise how tremendous an experience it is for your body, your mind, and your whole self to have this new way of being,…in the light of **managing** a different approach to your life,…with the ability you have to enjoy yourself in **everything** you do,…coupled with full confidence in the fact that you have accepted everything,… **you have ever experienced**, whatever it happened to be in the past,…it is now acceptable,…even something you can relish due to the learnings and teachings you gained from these experiences,…then all things considered,…I wonder if you can **fully enjoy** this new way of being,…celebrate it with a complete embracing, delightful **love**,…because when **you** do this,…you **will** automatically accept those boundless feelings of love that fold themselves all around your shoulders,…your head,…every part of your body,…keeping you safe,…comforted,…reassured,…

confirming your deepest beliefs and knowledge of the infinite love,…
and endless loving elements of all that is in, and comes into your
world right now,…helping you to **be** sure in the knowledge you
embody encompassing love,…being **all** good and **right** in every way,
…..

Next,…in your mind's eye,…take some steps towards the river,…
where there are ancient, majestic trees bending their branches in the
direction of the water,…which is flowing tunefully along,…
meandering over the pebbles and stones on the riverbed,…twisting
into myriad shapes and hypnotic patterns,…casting light and shade,
…ever changing as the constant flow moves relentlessly on its
journey to reach the sea,…during which time in this vision,…**you're**
standing by the riverside right now,…breathing in the clear fresh air,
…your body feels energised,…even powerful,…as if this walk has
been one of healing,…of reclaiming your full vitality,…where you
have **feeling**s of happiness **that** is connected to your wish to accept,
…**all** there is in the world and in the life around you,…where you are
enthused to accept,…and ultimately enjoy every single part of your
life that **has been** so far,… knowing you can do that right now,…as
you're **resolved** to sink deeper and deeper into the place of total
harmony,…the place of complete balance,…where you are indeed
the happiest,…feeling marvellous,…feeling peaceful,…feeling loving,
…with a sense of trust in your own self,…and your body and mind's
ability to resolve,…reorganise,…rejuvenate,…so that all within you
becomes serene and changed for the better,…how fabulous this
feels to you now,…just **recognise** and accept those feelings for a
few moments,…**your** inner **strength** to simply be **as** you are,…
without having to do anything other than let it happen,…you can be
sure **this** will happen,…that **is** certain,…as you listen to the sound of
my voice and all those **helpful** messages and suggestions the sound

of my voice brings **to you**, from the words I am saying, to the tone, the intonation,…**notice** the pace and even the volume of the words, as well as, the **words within words**,…in your mind's eye, turn **your** attention to the small boat moored a short distance away,…see **a** kind and **loving person** in the boat waiting to take you for a trip down stream,…to a place which is so **much more** in keeping with the way you like to be,…rather **than** the way life has caused you to be,…as you **just** allow **your body** to step onto this lovely boat,… then, feel the gentle rhythm of the buoyant floating nature of your journey,…**as** you enthuse about **all that you can** see on this trip,… as you **do** that,…you travel past relaxing, natural views of the countryside in its full abundance,…the leaves on the trees are lush, …with all shades of greens, browns, oranges, rich purples,…the grass **is** long,…interspersed with wild flowers of delightful colours,… **more** vivid and valuable, brighter **than bright**,…which holds **enough** of your attention as you pass by to maintain your feelings of awe and wonder,…whilst remaining comfortably calm and sleepy,…yet still, you are more and more relaxed,…falling comfortably and willingly into that state of transformation,…wherein your feelings can change for the better in all that you wish,…without having to do anything at all other than rest,…**be** placid, and simply let it happen,…for these reasons you feel **more** and more **in cooperation with** your willingness to accept,…more and more powerfully aware of all that unfolds, still quietly sure of your autonomy, of **your** ability to be mellow,…a **loving**, steady **self** in the best ways for you so that you have the most comforting experiences, from now on,…you can feel very pleased, even proud of this ability, that is so easy to tap into, **just** by letting go,…relaxing, **mov**ing your awareness **to** deep within you **where** there is found the peace and **harmony** which **is** yours to have,…and to use,…**bringing freedom** and autonomy,…keep hold of the love you have *for yourself*,…maintain compassion and complete understanding for all your life's journeys,…all of your experiences, knowing you are a loving caring being, a shining light, …when in your mind's eye *imagine* that *love* spreading from you all around your *being*,…at the same time it is *within* you,…touching those *you* love, *giving* them warm feelings of your *care and reassurance, as* if time does not exist,…*it's* a feeling of timelessness,…so you can take *all* the time *you need* to allow yourself,…as you **continue** to rest and relax,…to comfort those you love with the unbounded and infinite power of that love which is yours,…continue blending into the warm loving **accept**ance of your greater power and **love**, love that spreads beyond your body, even **as it** glows from you, it **is** expanding and **deepening**,…filling the space around you as well as **within you** with the most important element of who you are,…and **as** you do this, **you** can visualise your journey along the river is reaching the beach,…and the sea shore,… where you **feel** the air on your face change as a **clearer** fresher touch,…**like** an embrace of purity, a gentle stroke of your cheeks, **a** filling of clean air in your lungs, as you look around at the **bright** white and yellow sand on the empty beach,…contrasted with the turquoise of the ocean the imagine is **idyllic**,…spellbindingly **beautiful** so that as you take in slow deep **breath**s,…with your eyes closed for this, you feel the heat of the sun **which is** high in the sky, on your face,…on your hair and through your clothes,…**comforting**, refreshing your whole body **and** more importantly nourishing your feelings and thoughts,…so these become much **more agreeable,**… acceptable as a sense of serenity fills you with peaceful sensations all encompassing, at one with all that is,…you can hear beautiful music playing in your mind,…lifting your spirits, giving pleasure for as long as you desire this to be,…imagine **you're** laying on the hot soft sand,…still **enjoying** the heat of the sun's rays,…**resting** your body, allowing your mind to be still and quiet,…**in harmony** with your surroundings,…just letting all things be as they are, **so** you can fully be at one with all **that is good** for you at these very moments of being-ness and love,…and as you **stay peaceful**ly calm and relaxed you're falling into a welcome and pleasant sleep,…**which** is pleasant and **creates** a deeply transformational state of expansive love,…of **harmony** wherein you begin to dream the **most accepting**,…even magical dreams of wonder and awe **where you** are guided to reclaim your true self,…you **accept** abundance within **all** that you have seen and done throughout the days and weeks and months and years of **your learnings** and understandings,…where in this particular dream, those people you love so very much walk towards you as you lay on the sand,…sleeping and dreaming,… and they sit besides you, silently holding you, stroking your face, holding your hands,…then telling you adorable things about yourself that you had forgotten,…things that make you laugh, remind you of your goodness, reconnect you with the very best of yourself…………………

> At this point end the induction by bringing the client back to consciousness or allowing them to continue into sleep proper. If you prefer you can use the standard awakening script near the beginning of the book.

Induction for deep healing sleep

*This will take around half an hour when spoken carefully and slowly.
Begin by talking from this page first, then use standard physical relaxations 1 or 2
if further relaxation is needed.*

As usual, we begin by focussing on breathing. Ask the person to concentrate on their breathing. Breath with them for a while. Make sure the inward breaths are longer than the outward breaths. Try breathing in for seven counts, *one,.. two,.. three,.. four,.. five,.. six,.. seven,* then hold the breath for a count of three, then breath slowly out for a longer count,

one,..two,..three,..four,..five,..six,..seven,..eight,..nine,..ten,..more if possible. Repeat the breathing three times.

Next, if necessary to further relax the person, use a body scan relaxation for around five to ten minutes. See the methods at the beginning of the book, use relaxations 1 or 2, talking the person through the journey around their body, making adjustments where necessary depending on the physical health of the person you're working with. If someone has pain in a certain part of their body then avoid mentioning that area.

…..Let your thoughts follow the sounds of my voice,…and the rhythm the sound of my voice brings to you,…**accepting** the sense of **relaxation**,…and comfort that **comes** with letting go,…letting go of unwanted tensions,…**as you** follow the sounds and messages within my voice.

Be aware that your conscious mind can choose,…to **listen** to the messages within the sounds of my voice,…**with**in the tones and pace,…the inflections,….the **calm** tunes,…or your conscious mind can choose not to have **acceptance**,…listen to those messages and suggestions that help you to feel better,…with a sure sense **of** well being,…because your subconscious mind will,…always listen to **all** the helpful, healing messages,…within the **sleepy**, dreamy **sounds** of my voice that help you to,…find a place of safety, **here** within yourself,…**because** you will heal,…feel so much better in yourself,…**in** your thoughts and in **your** overall sense of health,…so that as we begin,…clear your **mind** of previous thoughts,…**you** now take three deeper breaths to **cleanse** your lungs and send oxygen around your body(*count the breaths with the person; one,…two,…three,…*),…just as **your thoughts** are becoming more and more dreamy,…**making** your muscles relax more and more,…as you allow **yourself** to sink into the surface beneath you,…**feel** a sense of increasing **comfort** and inner harmony,…**with** your body beginning to feel heavier,…**sleepier**,…in a good way,…so you can appreciate the truth, feeling **sensations** of how much you are deeply loved,…**as** you are indeed loved,…**you** are loved **unconditionally** and infinitely,…a universal love surrounds you,…**sink**s into you,…caresses you,…embraces you,….going **down** towards sleep,…without you having **to** do anything at all other than **rest** and relax,…so you can feel that love **right now**,…because the love is always there,…on every level of your being,…**you** can feel Love's presence so much more **easily**,…when you **sink** deeper and deeper **into** a wonderful state of **tranquility**,…finding peace,…and harmony,…knowing how much care and **understanding** there is for you,…**how** much pure loving energy,…**you can** heal,…and as you **drift** in your mind,…imagine right **now** at this moment you are being wrapped in **two** blankets of absolute loving **sleep**,…**where** the **warmth** and gentle tendernesses **within** that **love** comes to you and **holds you**,…keeping you safe,… just **as you're** so **sleepy**,…holding **your body** carefully with compassion,…as you choose to,…and your body **lets go**,…to sleep, …and **as you sleep**, follow the sound of my voice to a new place of being and cleansing,…drift down **deeper**, where only good can be found,…only strength,…strength **to** repair,…to reduce,…to **replenish yourself** with only good,…..now,…**in** this beautiful state of **deep relaxation**,…where **you are** enveloped in a quiet yet powerful healing,…loving,…enfolding,…imagine, as if **in a dream**,…you are walking through a forest lush and verdant,…with strong and magnificent trees, foliage, moss, undergrowth,…you're **walking** towards the clearing some way ahead,…and even though you're **asleep**,…there you can see this clearing in the distance,…**with every ambling step** you take **you are** moving nearer towards the sun beams shining onto the pathway,…**shining** onto the trees,…the leaves,…the branches,…the earth,…shining in straight lines,…**as if** pointing towards particular areas,…in the dense rich woodland,… moreover, the **drowsy** sunbeams draw you closer,…**yet** as **you** wish to get close to them,…you **imagine** they are **slumbering** rays of light,…guiding your journey out of the woods,…towards a clearer path,…**towards** fresh green fields lay ahead,,…where you will enjoy…a whole **new** environment,…another healthy, living **depths** of flora and fauna, which will,…lift your spirits,…giving you a gift **of** fresh, happier thoughts,…enjoyable feelings,…whilst in your **sleep** you're provided with panoramic views of astounding beauty,…as in time, right now,…as you enter the clearing,…that bright green space of lightness and clarity,…you can begin to **feel** the deepest of **relaxation** coming upon you,…just let go now, let go of unwanted physical tensions, more and **more**,…the peace and letting go seems to caress your body with **soothing** touches of love,…of kindness and absolute compassion,…for **yourself** and all which has transpired during your life,…**as you're** laying your body on the soft grass, enjoying the sensation of **letting go** of movement for a while, …you know you have arrived at a resting place filled with life and beauty,…it is there for you to enjoy,…for you to rest awhile,…**being reassured** of your right to be there,…to be **with** the grass on the ground, the surrounding tress,…there's pretty flowers nestling in the grass,…**thriving** bushes with red berries,…colourful birds playing in the undergrowth,…all whilst the sun continues its **restorative** often curative **intentions**,…diminishing unwanted physical feelings,… reassuring and repairing unwanted thoughts and behaviours,…you are **beginning** to imagine floating **dreamily** in**to** a mellow mesmerising **dream**,…a dream that in it's balmy serenity,…you can find restitution,…a pleasing freeing sensation that increases as you are soothed by all that surrounds you,……

You are **so** very **sleepy**,…completely tired,…**it** feels right for you to **allow** yourself to fall deeper and deeper into a wonderful dream filled **sleep**,…where your mind can comfort and console,…a mesmerising fabulous rhythmic sleep,…one of delicate dreams, creative dreams, …safe,…loving,…kind,…hushed and quiet, you drift down deeper and deeper, **realising** you have inner ability to find **restoration** of so much within you,…**is** so **right**, now sleep,…sleep,….deeper and deeper….

(if the person has fallen asleep here you may wish to let them sleep on and so you would not continue reading the script aloud. If you think they are still awake you can continue reading the words to the end of the transcript)….

In your dream you are aware of waking after a long sleep,…you are in the lovely clearing at the edge of the forest ,where all is good and pleasing,…and all your previous unwanted thoughts and feelings are forgotten,…lessened,….as can happen as **you sleep soundly** and well,…all manner of things have improved for you,… and you feel ready to continue on **your** journey out of the forest,…so imagine you are standing **quiet**, yet strong **and** tall, ready to walk forward,…to discover new and wholesome **tranquil** places,…that nourish, encourage,…even persuade your happiness and joy to emerge stronger,…giving consolation to your true self,….reconciling **your** uncertainties,…mediating with inner conflicts,…to provide resolutions and placation,….now, **fast**, as you look ahead, even though you're **asleep**, you see in the distance, a beach,…beyond the beach is a vivid turquoise sea,…which is so calm,…as you are deeper and deeper at **sleep**,…the water gently ebbing and flowing onto the white sand of the empty beach,…the view is **peacefully** idyllic ,…how clean and healthy the landscape appears to your eyes, …a delight to savour,…**so** astoundingly idyllic you take in a few **deep** breaths of awe and splendour,…the calming gentle breaths and the beautiful view makes you feel more **asleep**,…it has improved your conscious and subconscious thoughts,…you find you're more able to put **your** thoughts in order even when **drowsy**, …to wisely reconstruct some approaches of yourself **right now**,… you're reclaiming your true deepest self,…and this helps you to feel so much better,…in every way,…..and now,…even as **you're feeling lethargic** in your body,…in your mind's eye you're walking barefoot, strong and steady on the sun heated sand,..and you can feel the soft white sand between your toes,…feel the warmth of the sand welcoming you, comforting with every step you take,…**so sleepy**,… whilst the sounds of the waves as they gently ebb and flow are like music to your ears,…**somnolent**,…along with the seagulls in the sky above calling in their familiar way,…smell the salt air, the ozone,…just let yourself **drift into the deepest sleep**,…the freshness of pure natural sea air,…with all the healing, clearing abilities,…you can taste the salt on your lips, in your mouth, a good and healthy sensation that raises your spirits, energises you,…as you **stay sleepy,** feeling safe and comfortable,…because as you walk along the beach for some way,…there is no one there yet you are happy for it to be this way,…you're enjoying your own company,…enjoying all the sights and sounds around you,…noticing how at the same time, you're feeling so very **very sleepy**,…you lay down on the sand once more,…being drawn towards deep sleep, with your eyelids heavier and heavier,…as eventually you begin to feel so very,…**very tired**,…the most tired you have ever felt,…because as you heal all the parts of you that need and can be healed,…so you **feel** this very heavy **healthy tiredness** that takes you to a most satisfying, most welcome **sleep**,…as the sun pours down rays of benevolent heat which increases as it slowly reaches its highest point in the sky,…you are so hot,…in a good way,…more and more tired,…as you feel so much better in yourself,…the tiredness is a **good tiredness**,…one that informs you how good it is to **fall asleep** for as long as you need to,…knowing that when you awake you will be energised,…rested, feeling more optimistic, and ready to continue further on your journey,……

So for now, fall into that deep sleep, enjoy it,…sleep,…sleep,…deeper,…and deeper,…sleep.

If the person is not asleep that is absolutely fine, simply and quietly say to them that they can stay where they are for some moments and when they are ready they can open their eyes, stretch a little, then sit up, or take a sip of water.

Or if you wish, you can use the awakening script near the beginning of the book.

Feeling More Sure of Oneself

Use any standard relaxations inductions.

So lets begin...by allowing your physical body space and time,...to become still,...comfortable,...and relaxed,... in the knowledge,...that when your body relaxes,...totally and completely,...as you let go of unwanted physical tension in every cell of your body,......you will be much more able and willing,...to receive,...suggestions and ideas,...that are going to help **you**,...from now on,...to **feel** so much more sure of yourself,...in e**very** way,......furthermore,...in feeling so much more **sure** of your decisions,...**of** your thoughts and feelings,...you make changes within **yourself**,...within your thoughts, within your feelings, and in your behaviours,...that will cause you to feel so much more happiness,...because you will be living your life,...in the ways you wish,...and so for now,...all you have to do is listen,...to the words, sentences, to the suggestions the sound of my voice delivers to your subconscious mind,...and **let it happen**,...feeling increasingly relaxed,...as you continue listening to the sound of my voice,...so your physical body,...will certainly relax deeper and deeper,...taking the focus of your attention straight to your breath and your breathing,...so taking a deep breath in,...filling your lungs with air, when your lungs are full hold the breath for the count of five, ...1,2,3,4,5, and then very slowly, as slowly as you can,... breath out, ...then take in another deep breath, filling your lungs with air,...and hold the breath for the count of five 1,2,3,4,5,...and then slowly, slowly breath out, expelling the oxygen and all the waste products and toxins from your body,...as you continue breathing naturally and easily,...as **you** focus your attention now to the muscles in your feet and **make** your feet warm and soft, feel them becoming heavier and heavier,...more relaxed,...this relaxation feels **good**,...as it is a calming,...rejuvenating,...wholesome feeling,...like **decisions** you've made that work out well,... as the relaxation is spreading now into your ankles,...and your ankle muscles are becoming more calm, ...still,...so that **feel**ing spreads to your calves and your shins,...and it's a quiet **confidence** that you feel as your body listens to your mind and relaxes,...its a good feeling,... a warm and full feeling,... softness,...looseness,...simply letting all your muscles be,...in that comforting state,...of calm and harmony,...whilst the feeling spreads to your hips,...all around your hips,... softer,...letting go,...letting be, ...your stomach muscles relaxing,...as **you** breath easily and naturally,...your subconscious and your conscious mind are listening to the sounds and the words my voice makes,...to help you **feel** and become the way you **sure** wish to be,...for the better,...as the muscles **of** your back relax more and more and you're feeling heavier and heavier **all** over,...your chest, your clavicle and shoulders,...**your** shoulder blades, and the rest of your body makes the **decision s**taying calm and relaxed,...staying peaceful,...your upper arms, elbows and lower arms now are feeling heavier,...loose and limp and soft,...your hands the upper hands the palms of your hands,...your thumbs and fingers,...just at peace,...in tune with the calmness, that is throughout **your** body,...and spreading into your neck muscles,...feeling your neck muscles **settling** and sinking into a wonderful,...beautiful place of tranquility,...and feeling the weight of your head as it rests against the surface beneath it,...you notice the whole of your body has become so much more at ease,...and will continue to do so as **you** listen to the sound of my voice,... because it's a good feeling, when you **can** remain so calm,...and your conscious mind can **easily** choose to listen to the sound of my voice,…and the helpful messages that the suggestions in the sound of my voice brings to you,…or your conscious mind can **decide** not to listen to the sounds of my voice, thats absolutely fine,…because **in** fact your subconscious mind will listen constantly to **all** the sounds of my voice,…and all the helpful messages and suggestions the sound of my voice brings to you in all **situations**,…and your subconscious mind feels confident knowing the validity of all those helpful messages and suggestions that will change the way **you** are, …for the better,…creating inner joy, happiness, and a sense of well being,…so you can reliably relax to **enjoy** more and more,…knowing your subconscious mind will take control,…**choosing** which changes will happen,…from now into your future,…**as** all you have to do is accept and rest and relax,…**doing** nothing but letting go of any residual unwanted tension,…**so** whilst in your mind's eye imagine you're walking along a path,…where happiness **causes** you to amble comfortably,…this path is in a picturesque forest where the sun is shining above,…warming **you**,…making the atmosphere balmy,…when you look **to** the right,…you can see and **feel** the trunks of the trees with gnarled bark,…where birds are **secure**ly nesting in holes **and** in the **safe**ty of branches high up,…then you smell the humid dense aroma of woodland,…and when you look up you see branches and leaves forming a canopy over the forest,… and **you** feel wholesome,…you **feel** a conviction that you are doing the right thing to walk along the path,…giving yourself **positive** constructive time to think **and** make absolute decisions,…then next you **choose** to look to the left where **the** trees are very beautiful but more sparse, so you can **best** see the undergrowth and clearings **of** the forest,…giving assurance,…that **all** the wildlife,…is healthy and strong,…with resources to maintain their wellbeing,…and your **option's** to walk along comfortably and happily for some time,…

being certain that at some point soon the path,...***is*** about to split into two,...and for you it's ***delightful*** to choose whether to follow the path on the right or to follow the path on the left,...so ***as*** you prepare yourself to make that decision,...all the while enjoying the heat and balmy weather,...feeling ***well***,...breathing in the sweet rich smells of the forest,...***as*** you feel the twigs and moss underneath your feet with each light and ***easy*** step you take,...as well as, from time to time,...***you*** hear the rustle to the left in the undergrowth where small animals scamper from one place to another,...then with bold steps and ***feel***ing self reliance,...keep walking, you're ***happier***, gathering strength and determination ***now*** as ***you*** walk,......you ***are*** seeing the path split into two paths, the path on the right meanders ***more*** into the forest,...out of sight,...whereas the path to the left,...is more straight and ***sure***, taking you away from the forest towards fields and green hills,...so you stand wondering shall I take the path to the right or shall I take the path to the left

,...appreciating ***you*** will reach a conclusion,...after making judgement,...in placing reliance on your ability to consider options,...and so trusting in your own wisdom,...you ***feel*** confident in your choice,...***accepting***,...you've made the right ***choice***,...at the right time,...***is*** for the **right** reasons,...because you decided,...sensibly and ***rationally***,...knowing that at any point,...after walking down whichever path you've chosen,...you may choose new decisions in the future,...and so ***you*** feel so positive,...***hav***ing faith in your abilities,...and walking along the path you've ***chosen*** you notice how with each step you take,...***and*** you ***are*** feeling much more at one with yourself,...***happy***,...moreover you've gained energy,...and as that happens,...***you*** to feel resolute,...with increased ***trust*** in ***yourself***,...having discovered,...how to be precise,...and exact,...in any circumstances,...so you continue your amiable, health giving walk,...all the while observing the landscape around you,...until you are ready to rest and relax into your comfortable decisions,...more and more,...feeling so much better in each and every way,...

> At this point end the induction by bringing the client back to consciousness or allowing them to continue into sleep proper. If you prefer you can use the standard awakening script near the beginning of the book.

Healing River *to promote health*

use any of the preliminary inductions before starting this healing script

So let's take one deep breath in,…hold it,…and then very slowly release that breath,…and another deep breathe in,…hold it,…and slowly breathe out,…that's good,… and now continue breathing easily and naturally,…feeling the warmth of your body,…from the flow of energy that travels around your body,…knowing that with each breath you breath in you're breathing in clean fresh air,…that travels to your lungs and then is taken all around your body,…in your veins, cleaning, clearing, hearing, restoring each and every cell of your body,…so **you** gain strength,…gain a deeper forms of energy,…which **are** the life force of your organic self,…as it heals and restores,…giving you **much** more power,…and when you breathe out, you feel so much **better**,…as you're breathing out the toxins,…**and** the waste products,…calming and soothing **your** body,…and this process of breathing in and breathing out is continuous,…**healing**,…soothing,…calming,…caring,…**every** single **part** of you,..as you rest and relax in **each moment**,…encouraging your body to let go of unwanted tension,…feeling your body becoming softer,…the muscles are loose,…you can relax more and more,…..

Listening to the sounds of birds, and imagining that **you're** sitting by the side of a beautiful river,…your **thoughts** are calm ones,…as the river gently meanders along,…you **are** peaceful, with a sense of stillness,…**so** as you look into the river,…you see it's deep enough for rowing boats,…for **positively** all types of steam boats,…small

powered boats,…**and** all around there's lush green grasses and wild flowers,…and **you** can **hear** the sound of the birds as they **are** singing freely,…not **only** in the trees,…where there are many **lovely** birds to see,…but some of them have their branches leaning into the river water,…**useful** cascading canopies,…and there are so many different colours of green,…in the foliage, the plant life,…this is all **new** to you,…in a good way,…giving you new ideas and helpful **messages**,…and all is quiet apart from the sound of the water in the river,…which is meandering towards the sea in the far far distance,…and the birds of all varieties,…of countless colours and shapes,…singing their songs.,,, the sun is shining in the sky,…pouring down it's heat and it's rays,…and that heat and those rays,…penetrating into you through **your** clothes,…giving you vitality,…and a pure life force of the earth,…**transforming**,…changing clearing creating health,…wellbeing of **yourself**,…a boat drives up,…to the water's edge,…it's a small boat powered by a motor,…and the person who's driving it steps out,…walks into the distance,…**continuing** on their journey and the boat is there for you **to** use,…and as you step into this boat you **notice** the river is quite murky,…muddy,…cloudy,…and between **the** mud and the cloudiness,…when you looking the water you can see fishes swimming below,…which is a **good** thing,…and you sit comfortably **in** the boat,…**everything** is in your control,…holding the steering lever,…and then allow one your arms to drop into the water,…so **you** can **feel** the warm temperature,… then as you splash with your hand the water clears easily and **well**,…just around where you put **your** hand into the water,…it's **remarkable**,…there's a small circle of fresh clean water,…and **because** when you look into it **you can** see the fish and underwater plant life,…on the bed of the river,…so you **appreciate the importance** that this happened simply by you being there and placing your hand in the water,…as this is a special type **of healing**,…one that you have within you,…to do this with **yourself**,……

so now start the boat,…with a key or a lever,…and the engine starts,…powered by the sun,…and you steer the boat gently down the river,… whilst you enjoy the warm breeze,…on your face and through your clothes,..as you breath deeply,…because it's such a good feeling to you,…to fill your lungs full of clean fresh air,…refreshing your mind,…clearing your thoughts,…you want to smile,…you feel so happy,…and you notice, when you turn around and look at where you've been,…that as you've moved down the river,…with your hand at the helm,…**all** the water around you is clean,…and the murkiness has disappeared,…and you can see the pebbles at the bottom **of** the river bed,…there's something about you being there,…**this** is important indeed,…as it **means** you have the power and the strength to cleanse the river,…there is something about **you** and the boat,…**are** making the journey,…that has tremendous power to change nature,…**healing** it for the better,…and on the banks of the river as you cast your eyes you can see beautiful sights of,…wild animals **such** as beavers,…**with strength** and fortitude, busy making dams,…water voles, red squirrels,…**and** colourful birds,…of all varieties,…its as if they've all **joyful**ly congregated to be near you,..the cardinals from Kentucky,…the toucans from South America,…parrots,…and all other gorgeous birds you are **resolve**d to see,…they are there,…swans,…ducklings and ducks, the male and the female duck **promoting** the little duckling following behind,…the **health**y geese flying above,…colourful pheasants,…the loud peacocks,…white doves,…along with all nature and native birds,…so magical,…the field mice popping up,…hedgehogs,…and salmon jumping out of the water then back in again,…all the while the wild flowers continue blooming and blossoming stronger,…gently blowing in the wind,…a little further on,…you see a barge,…moored by the side of the riverbank,…and you pull up behind it,…turn off the engine,…step out of your boat, onto the barge,…and there inside **your** family await,…smiling,…happy,…**looking so well**,…just **as** you look so well,…all filled with **energy and joy**,…because this **is** a hand made extraordinary barge,…when **you're** sailing it,…**purpose**fully,…someway ahead,…there is a country pub,…for your lunch,…**and** you can take your time getting **there**,…enjoy being **in** the barge,…looking in the cupboards,…**all** clean,…filled with useful **things** to help you on your journey,…**for** it's such fun,…just enjoy your time **now**,…there in the barge,…feeling the buoyancy in the water,…**feel**ing the transformation of the river,…seeing **how** clean the water is,…and how you have **improved** the wildlife,…**you are** amazing,…**in every way**,…and over time,…which has been wonderful,…you reach the country pub by the side of the riverbank,…where you can,…step inside,… it is rustic with history,…and delightful,…spend time there,…nourishing your bodies,…sharing thoughts and ideas,…happy and positive,…as that sense of health strength and vitality,…continues,…and improves and develops,…from now,…onwards into the future,…

> At this point end the induction by bringing the client back to consciousness or allowing them to continue into sleep proper. If you prefer you can use the standard awakening script near the beginning of the book.

Induction for health anxiety/conflict resolution/inner peace

Use one of the standard relaxation inductions 1, 2, 3 or 4.

…..and imagine right now,…..as you walk along,….barren and dusty terrain, you're carrying all the burdens with you that,.. you feel,…in your life right now,…and when **you** look to the left,…you **can** see barren, desert, dry, landscape, flat and uninspiring, occasional dusty bushes close the ground,…it all **become**s dryer the further away you look,…and when you look to your right,…you see a **calm** dry flat, dusty landscape stretching far into the distance onto the horizon…..as you **look ahead** the dust and the sand and the heat has created a haze,…so **your vision** sees a distorted,…almost wobbly scene of dry dusty terrain,…which **is becoming** hotter and dryer,…no **clearer**,…and yet you walk oblong the path because that is the direction **you** are impelled to walk… forward one step after another,…and you **realise** those burdens **you** carry are heavy,…and there are many,…..and walk carefully, as you **can** trip over the dry bush close to the ground,…it feels so hard when the landscape doesn't **change** so you sit on the ground **for** a while,…taking **the** time to breath more deeply,…which feels **better**,…and lets breath in now,…a big deep breath **and** then hold it,…one, two, three, four, five,…then very slowly breath out,…as slowly as **you** can,…that's good,…and **keep** your eyes still closed breath in one more time a big deep breath, filling your lungs with air, one, two, three, four, five, **the** breath is slowly releasing, **change**,…ing your state of being,… helping you feel calm,…as long as it takes to clear the air **from** your lungs,…and **now** breath naturally,…and easily, from now **on**,…that's good,…and when you look inside in your mind's eye the landscape has changed somewhat,…whereas before,…when you looked to the left you saw **all** your problems,…affecting **your previous** thoughts and feelings,…and when you looked to the right you looked over the **concerns** and difficulties from others,……you **have** noticed,…as you look ahead now,…the landscape has changed,…the haziness has **gone**,…**and** if you look carefully,…there in the distance,…**you** can see a bright green field,…you **feel** a sense of hope in this new landscape,…the sun is still **strong** and hot in the sky,…nourishing the grass,…just laying between the problems on the left and the issues and difficulties on the right,…**with a** sense of hope and **confidence**,…flowers are growing lush and verdant,…standing tall and **sure** in the field **of** emerging new life,…and now,…gathering **yourself** together,…you walk to this field,…this is called the field of impartiality,…where there is only peace,…tranquility,…harmony,… you experience good feelings when you go there,…go there now, …..**you've gained** so much balance and **peace**,……see the beauty in all that is in this field,…flowers of all colours,…violets, reds, purples, blues, yellows, whites,…and **with** vivid greens of many shades and smell the **innate** freshness from the plant life,…bringing **happiness and joy** as you step onto the soft welcoming grass,…it's as if the field expands,…you can see the land ahead **full of** lush verdant expanse,…growing stretching,…**continuing**,…filling the whole of your vision with **good** and natural beauty,…**health** giving,… beneficial,…everywhere you look,…**all** around,…you are calmed,… you find **the** inner peace,…that lifts your spirits,…at just this right **time**,…and provides you with the **right** inner nourishment,…right **now**,…giving you well-being,…and steadfast love **for** yourself,…and as you look to **the** left you see the **rest of** the landscape is fields beyond fields,…**your** feelings are uplifted,…fields of sheep and lambs, full of **life**,…beautiful flowers and long grass,… the birds are flying high in the sky,…and beyond that you see rolling hills,…with trees dotted on their slopes,…and the sky is beautiful blue,…with a few wispy clouds,…and this stunning landscape fills your vision,…there's a long, winding path **you're** standing on,….meandering away onto the line of the horizon,…as far as your eye can see,…and to the right there is **beautiful** dense rich forest,..a number of different types of trees,…their trunks,…some are gnarled and ancient,…. others are new and fresh and straight,…and their branches and leaves are forming a canopy,…of shade,…and beyond that **you** can hear the movement of water,…somewhere beyond the forest you'll **find** a river or stream with waterfalls,…and **you can** hear the birds from within,….the birds within the branches of the trees,…you can see them flying in the sky,…whilst the sun is delightfully hot,…helping you **resolve**,…feel healed,…soothed,…**all** loving,…kind,…nurturing reassurance,…that everything is so much better now,…so accept **your** new feelings,…and those of comfort and reassurance,…removing **conflicts**,…allowing acceptance and harmony to permeate your whole being,…allowing you to revel in the sure knowledge you have connected to your true inner self,…that is good,…**with** a sense of kindness and enjoyment,…in being at one with **yourself**,…with nature,…**and** feeling positive life all around you,…providing you **with** renewed energy and joy,…as you gladly left **other s**adnesses behind in the barren landscape,…with all those unwanted thoughts and feelings,…they've become unnecessary, irrelevant, faded into the background,…**because** it is time for **you** to rediscover,…inner strength,…knowing your subconscious mind will resolve all those unwanted issues,…you feel so much happier now,…**find** stillness,…because your feelings are in tune with your real deeper self,…so you continue to feel **inner** steadfast resilience,...as you stand in your field of impartiality,...noticing right now,...there is a gentle, wise person waiting at the edge of the field to guide you towards **joy**,...because this is your new journey,...of connection,...to your true self of health **and** wellbeing,...where you gather **resources** to create a new way forward,...and this person in the field of impartiality,...takes you,...to happiness,...contentment,...joy...so **that** you find only goodness within,...as well as love,...and kindness,...because it is always possible to be here,...as you **are** dreaming or think **deep**ly, or simply relax and let it happen,...**and** you keep this close to the surface as you go about your living daily experiences,...you walk towards this person who is **effective** in helping you,...and notice how truly wise and kind the person is...you can see it **in** their eyes and in their stature and emanating from them is a sense of love,...**all** welcoming and accepting,...as they know you so well,....and are willing and ready to guide you in all **circumstances** and help you to **maintain** full enjoyment,...within your lived **experience**,...then together you walk into the forest,...on the path between the trees **and** the undergrowth,...when with each step you take you gain **energy**,...as your guide talks words of wisdom that helps you completely remove unwanted issues you left behind,...whilst all you have to do is **enjoy** the walk, allowing **the** words to **flow** into you without having to do anything at all other than listen to **let it** happen, ...taking in the rich damp smell of the forest,...go towards the undergrowth and the myriad lives living there,...the smallest insect **or** the largest deer,...**let** each one feel like a gift,...**it**'s because you're in tune with yourself,...you can **be** happy,...whilst your whole being is transformed for the better,...then after some time,...the path guides you both out of the forest,...to a clearing,...where you can see to the left rolling hills beyond the fields,...in addition there is a dusty path stretching all the way to the hills,…next, your kind, wise and loving guide indicates it's time to walk along this path alone,…towards the hills the distance,… and **you** do that happily, with confidence,…moreover, from time to time rabbits hop in front of you showing no fear,…as they know you are safe, you **will** show kindness, **be** loving, they feel it,…as do the dragonflies and butterflies,…and the birds,…all **happy**,…eventually, a female deer steps onto the path,…indicating through movement she is going to guide you for the rest of the journey toward the hill,…**you can** touch her fur speckled so soft as you touch her you **feel**,…in your hand and through your arms, through your whole body the gentle **pure love** that is this deer,…she walks slowly at your pace,…in tune,…**with your** inner **self** and you can feel within you,…opening up of your inner essence,…besides strengthening your resolve,…you're gaining power of all kinds,…eventually,….you reach the foot of the hills,…where you see a quaint and pretty cottage,….with a walled garden, with roses over the door,…also beautiful flowers in the front garden,…furthermore,…the front door is open,…realising this is your cottage,…which belongs to you,……so it's **your** place of **safe**ty,…where you find balance,…to retreat to gather yourself, gaining strength in all ways,…as you do that right now,…walking up the path to the front door then stepping inside,…where you will be able to take time,…to take stock,…wherein all within you can be still as you celebrate the reemergence of your inner serenity and all that is good, …

> At this point end the induction by bringing the client back to consciousness or allowing them to continue into sleep proper. If you prefer you can use the standard awakening script near the beginning of the book.

Overcoming Pain

Use a standard physical relaxation.

…………You can imagine,…right now,…you are standing…..at the entrance of your…inner garden….which is expansive and full of life….of flowers,…trees,.. bushes,…so many colours of green,…so many fragrances,….and… when **you** are standing in your garden,…as you are…right now…you **feel** contented,…a **happiness** comes upon you,…even though,..there is much work to be done in this garden of yours,..to,..make it beautiful and healthy,… more organised….

It's as if winter's over,…spring has arrived,..and all the life,..of each and every plant…is sprouting and bursting,..growing and its time **now** to **control** your garden,…because **you'r**e in charge,…and you will make it the most bountiful,…colourful,…fragrant,..delightful,..**health**iest garden,..for the whole of the spring,..the summer,..the autumn,..right into the winter,..and in order to **do that**,..right now,…imagine,…as if its absolutely real,..that **you** pick up a watering **can**,..to revive the plants that need moisture,…then **get** some gardening tools,…so that you can **better**,..tidy up the garden,…**and**,…now..it's time,..to start to **remove all** the weeds,..and all **unwanted** junk,..that is lying around your garden…..it's hard **physical** work, but you're happy to work hard,…because as a result of your hard work the real **changes** are all around,…there for the future **for** everyone to see…You feel **full** of pride for the work you've done,..and for the work you'll continue to do…the garden's looking **health**ier,…more wholesome,..and tidy,…**where**,..before there was chaos,... *you* realise,...that you *are*... the one who has masterminded the *successful* completion and transformation of your beautiful garden.

And,.. *you can*,..breath deeply,..allowing yourself to *continue*,..to imagine the shape,..and the colours,..and the style,..the *pleasure* of your garden....this garden that belongs to you is magic,...its a magical garden,...and...you are aware that *the* plants in this magic garden remove *pain*...so,..you decide which of the plants *is* the best for you,...so,...hold some of those wonderful magic plants,..and after you've *removed* them *from* the ground,...immediately *your* whole self *senses*,...a lightness,..a freeing,..clarity,..a sense of healing,..*so* holding the plants carefully,..lovingly,..*you* place them in water where they *are* sure to thrive,..all the while being *aware* of a natural mildness,..and softening,..in yourself in your feelings,..and in your being,..*and* continue reorganising the rest of your garden,...........
just *notice* how easy it is to create,... *how* pleasant looking and *much better* the garden looks,...and *you* can *feel*,.. through your creativity,..determination,..hard work,...you continue to *do that*... finding happiness and joy....as you allow the garden to take shape,..knowing deep within you *you* are right,..to refine all the greenery,...all the plant life,..because it changes the way you *feel*, ...so now you are *comforted*,...and you can bathe *in* the sunny congenial,..lush olive groves,..*a* bonus are the olives found on the tree,..by the waterfall...which is pouring *gentl*-y into the pond,..creating a steam like *haze* above the water.. along with the pleasing sounds... *of* fluid cascades,..providing you with *happiness* and joy..

So *you* can *feel proud* of yourself for all the work you have done... all the while...feeling more free,..and more comfortable,..more at one,..and able to rise above all but acceptable feelings,….because in this deep state of relaxation….**you are** able to transform….all things within you,…for the **good** and the better,..for health and wellbeing… just as you are able to reject all things not for good,…all negative aspects,…**you can** rectify or eject….just as in your garden you can eliminate the unwanted plants or weeds,..and you dismiss and **clear away** overgrown areas…branches….so you can do that…within your own self….deflating and receding,..creating….a dwindling to nothing..of **unwanted elements**…..because within your garden sometimes you feel it is awful how untidy it is,..and how messy,…you can change it *now,*….as you do so you will,..notice how you **feel** lighter,..**free**,..a sense of safety and clarity that is manifest within you,…a lightness of being,..**which** is reliable and constant….and **for you**,..you find this **is controllable** and you can keep those pleasant feelings,..**whilst** eradicating the unwanted….you've worked so hard **in** your garden,.the **time** has come to be restful,..as **you find** a sunny spot where you can sit,..perhaps in a sun lounger or a chair or even lay down on the grass,..graceful..and **peace**ful…such a satisfying feeling to enjoy the bounty of your hard work….and **within** you,..you feel glowing a sense of natural health….and there will be times **now**,..as you drift into deeper,..and deeper,..sleep,..where you will not be aware of your body,….you wont be aware of your body at all,…as you continue to go deeper and deeper,…relaxed,.. deeper,..and deeper,..and deeper….

> At this point end the induction by bringing the client back to consciousness or allowing them to continue into sleep proper. If you prefer you can use the standard awakening script near the beginning of the book.

Withstanding fear

start with relaxation induction number 3....

So now,…**you are** going to, remove all that unwanted fear and anxiety,..all the unnecessary tensions,…the thoughts and the behaviours,…that create so much difficulty,…replacing them with **strong** thoughts and feelings,…..and in order to begin, remember you are safe,…**you** can manage this,……so ensure you have a quiet place where you can **feel** calm,…remaining uninterrupted and at **peace** with yourself for at least half an hour,…**always** ensure your clothing is loose and that your body is free from tightness,…at the same time **your** limbs are straight and not crossed,…your neck is **comfortable**,…whether you're laying down or sitting,…**and** we'll begin your journey to peace, **calm** and harmony,…by using the breath,…because if we breath steadily with purpose,…**you** can change the state of your physical body,..and improve,…the rhythms and the chemicals that are released from our brains,…so we will **feel** so much more tranquil, calm, **courageous**,…and rested,…sure of ourselves,…on the deepest of levels,…to get **ready**, take in one slow, deep breath and hold that breath for the count of five,…one, two, three, four, five,…release,…breath out more slowly than the speed **to** which you breathed in,…then again, **accept** the in breath slowly, steadily as you fill your lungs.

Hold for a count of five,…one, two, three, four, five,…then breath **all** the air out,…so much more slowly,…and one more time in this same **situation**, **s**o breath in, fill your lungs, hold for five,…one, two, three, four, five,…and then breath out very very slowly, and **easily**,…..that's good, well, let's continue,…**regardless of** external sounds,…focus your body **whatever** else **they** may signal,…as you **are** continuing to breath easily and steadily,…**so** you're breathing,…in a rhythmical manner,…quite naturally as **you** focus on your body and any tightnesses in your muscles around your body,…and to do that you **are** taking the focus of your attention to the muscles within the soles of your feet,…allowing those muscles to become softer,…**feeling** more loose,… feel the warmth,…spreading as comfort into your toes, …the whole of your feet,…you have **determination** as the whole of your feet become softer, more relaxed, all the while breathing steadily,…because **through** that,….you will slowly and surely feel much more safe,…**which** is much more comfortable,…a steadiness coming upon **you** and a resolve,…as that feeling of relaxation **will** move into your ankles, into your calves and your shins,….filling them with peace and harmony,…as you **overcome unwanted** tensions,… the **idea is** it's feels like a loving, soothing caress,…**or** a **real** caring tender touch,…**experiences** of gentle pleasure,…moving **easily**, lovingly into the backs of your knees,…**and** your thighs,…your hips…calming,…**naturally** comforting,..its a loving sensation,… gentle delicate,…yet powerful….and that feeling is spreading now,… into your stomach,…your lower back,…erasing the tension,…**just** using power of your mind as you focus on **let**ting go and softening,… creating a safe space,…**it** will **happen**,……drifting,…increasingly,… into a serenity,…**without** effort,…your chest,…your middle and upper back,…as **you** sink into the surface beneath you,…**having** comfort,…**to** know you are safe,…to **do anything** at all,…**only** all is well,…**allow** yourself to feel as if you can float,…whilst relaxing **your** muscles,..so **subconscious mind** can help you,…just as your shoulders relax,…your clavicle,…**to** your shoulder blades,…**take** that gentle loving energy,…to your upper arms and elbows,…letting go of **control** of your lower arms,…**bringing** harmony to your wrists,

...moving **forward** to the backs of **your** hands,...the **inner** palms of your hands,...your thumbs and fingers,...a lightness of **power**,...**to** feeling so much more comfortable,...to **resolve**,... **and** letting **go** more and more,..breathing steadily,..gently,...going **forward**,... sensitively,...**as** your neck muscles feel **a** relaxing relief,...then a **new** feeling is your head is pressing into the surface beneath it,... **and** this feels **better**,...the welcome weight of your head resting and relaxing more and more,......this **version of** relaxation is deep and powerful,...let go of any residual tension within **yourself**,...the muscles underneath your scalp,...as underneath your hair,...**right** up to the crown of your head you can feel the muscles there relaxing, ...you can feel the muscles round your eyes relaxing,...and **now** the muscles in your forehead softening,...it's as if someone is softly stroking your head,...with love,...with care,...**from** tenderness and attention,...**now** the muscles behind your eyebrows are softening,... **you're** loosening,...your eyes are **much** more still, as if asleep,... and your eyelids are closed,...your cheeks **more** warm and full,... you feel nourished, yet calmly **adventurous** to continue relaxing,... your tongue loose inside your mouth, **showing** complete letting go, ...as if, now, your body is engulfed by loving, caring, **tenacious** attention,...with **qualities** to soothe,...support,...guide and,...**in** relaxing you, this feeling will continue,...**all** the time, as it is infinite,... simply by thinking in this way in all **situations** you will feel safer,... protected,...loved,...unconditionally,...and cared for because it seems **as** if your body now feels so heavy,...**you** can sink into the surface beneath you as a relief,...and in this place of restoration,... and of rejuvenation,...you can **gain** strength within you,...because the resolve and resilience is natural,...without your **self** having to do anything at all,...other than let it happen,...**value** this ability,...as you realise,...it is also as if in,...another way,...you're feeling lighter than air,…like you could float upwards,…five to ten centimetres above your current resting place,…feel that now,…and **enjoy that** sensation,…of being lighter than air,…the ability to float in whichever ways you choose,…but for now,…allow yourself to drift back down to your original resting place there,…so that,…..in **your** minds eye,…as you imagine you're sitting on a white fine sandy beach alone,…comfortably so,…your **energy levels** are still and focussed,…you're in this place of reflection,…rejuvenation,…**increas**ingly a place of recovery,…you are looking out,…over a turquoise ocean,…**with** waves slowly, gently ebbing and flowing,…**a sense of** repetition,…the sun pouring down healing rays of warmth,…**a** welcome **joy**ful energy,…majesty,..**and** power,…increasing **satisfaction** as you sit looking out over the turquoise water, the blue sky,…where occasional seagulls fly past briefly **changing** the view,…you can taste the salt from the ocean on your lips,…and smell the ozone and the clear fresh air,…all **unwanted feelings** have disappeared,…you can feel the dry white sand between your fingers,…as you filter it through **into** the palms of your hands,…creating an **exhilarating** feeling within you,…realise, right now as your **energy** calms and comforts,…how your conscious mind can choose to listen to the sound of my voice,…and the helpful messages and suggestions the sound of my voice brings to you,…or your conscious mind can choose not to,…listen to the sound of my voice,…that's absolutely fine,…because your subconscious mind will listen to all the messages and suggestions the sound and tone of my voice brings to you that are,…going to help **you**,…from now on to,…feel so much better,…in your thinking,…and in **have**ing better feelings,…and the ways you react with **courage**,…and behave in your day to day life……………….

In your state of calm and relaxation and always,…each time I use the word 'now',…just like that, 'now' **you** will fall deeper and deeper into a place of loving,.…peaceful,..harmony, where you **have** transformative shifts slowing down,…for the better,…from now on,…you can do that as you,…rest and relax, whilst maintaining inner **strength**,…and allow yourself to drift along,…without having to do anything other than,…be yourself,…as you will find resolve and resilience within you,…moreover,…since you continue to find comfort,…rest,…harmony,…balance and tranquility within the images **you** create,…and the suggestions my voice brings to you,…as you **are** looking out across the ocean,…feeling more like your usual healthy, **resolute** self you see in the distance,…the far,…far distance,…a sailing boat on the horizon,…slowly making its way from one place to another,…whereas as you look up into the clear blue sky there is a small dot,…which must be a magical bird, flying towards you with intention,…with power and might,…and as it flies nearer and nearer **you can** identify it,…it is an enormous, benevolent eagle flying in to help you,..…flying to the beach,…the bird **settles down** close to you,…and when you look into his eyes they are filled,…with compassion and consolation,…the bird brings with it an,…energy of understanding,…of dedication to you,…during which,…**you** understand,…from the movement of the bird's majestic, …magnificent,…head that,…you will **gain confidence**,…from him,…he is inviting you to alight on his back,…and **because** you trust his ability to help you,…**you do that**,…hold your arms around his neck **whilst** he spreads his enormous wingspan and begins to move the wings **powerfully** up and down, gracefully,…with rhythm,…and you're **lifting** up into the sky,…feeling the wind on your cheeks and through **your** hair,…its exhilarating and empowering,…and you can, feel sensations of **happiness**,…a new joy,…and the higher you fly,…

the more you see,…as you look at the beach below and the ocean, the sand dunes,…then,…further away fields and towns, road and cities,…mountains,…**higher and higher** you fly,…all the **while feeling stronger** and stronger,…a sense of restitution,…is coming upon you,…residing within you,…**amidst** invigoration,…restoration, …meanwhile,…you fly high enough to reach some wispy white clouds,…firm, **solid** clouds on which the eagle rests a while,…and you dismount and walk around,…these are called the clouds of **knowing**,….where you can,..take stock of all you know and that has been,…without having to really think **about** all that,…just let it happen,…at the same time feeling provided with inner **wisdom and power**,….

This is a place,…of silence,…with energy,…giving unconditional infinite love,…and you enjoy feeling the energy nourishing you on every level,…and,…after some time you climb onto the eagle, holding tight as he takes you higher and higher,…so high you can see whole continents down below,…and still **you feel strong**,…able, … gaining and reclaiming,…energy more than that,…a sense of justice alongside acceptance,…and eventually,…you reach some dense white,…snow white,…clouds, where the eagles rests,…once again,…as you dismount a lightness within your being,…washes over you like a wave,…wherein you,…accept the beauty and the splendour,..of all you can see as well as all that has been,…these are the clouds of unknowing,…there is so much there for you to help you as it soaks into you,…you can combine all that is there,….,into your essence,…here,..you rest for quite some time…where **you feel better**,…your creative self developing,…healing,……………..

then the time is right to climb upon the eagles back as he carefully flies down towards the earth,…and you can see,…as you descend further and further that the beach is in sight,…including the beautiful ocean, glistening with the suns rays upon it,…and eventually he lands gently on the fine white sand,….and you dismount,..thanking the bird for his tremendous journey,…his gift to you,…and lay your self on the sand,…as you sit there you watch him open his wings once more then fly away in the direction he came from,…as **you**,…all the while,…**are**,…**feeling peaceful**,…yet powerful,…consoled,…moreover,…you are tired,…so you lay on the sand resting your head and the whole of you body,…closing your eyes, breathing steadily,…feeling a warm sensation throughout the whole of your body,…and **you're so relaxed**,…feeling so much good has come,…through this journey,…you're falling into a deep,…soothing,..caressing,…loving,…healing sleep,…sleep,…knowing that as you sleep,…all is well,..and all is safe,…furthermore you begin to dream,..a transformational dream,…of restoration and vitality,…dreaming on the deepest of levels,..where you find,..serenity,…calm,…and you sleep so deeply,…you dream of wonder,….dreaming more than that,…you are sitting on a white fine sandy beach,…the beach is empty,…apart from your self and you feel rested relaxed,…comforted and comfortable,…so sleep,..sleep…sleep…

> At this point end the induction by bringing the client back to consciousness or allowing them to continue into sleep proper. If you prefer you can use the standard awakening script near the beginning of the book.

Coping with illness, increasing well being

Begin with relaxation, number 1 or 2.

Remove from *your* mind all thoughts except those of safety,… wellness,…and love,…as you remind yourself of the transforming **strength** you have,…to change so much within yourself,…from your sense of inner power,…to your thoughts,…as well your feelings,…as it all **becomes** the transformative energy that can make all the difference - for the **greater** good,…so that as you listen to the sound of these words,…allow yourself to gently sink into the comfort of the …. (*cushions, pillows, settee, duvet, whatever the person is resting on*)… and **feel** your body simply letting go,…of unwanted tensions, …of tightness within muscles,…being aware of movements in *your body*,…wherever they are,…just notice that,…as your mind **lets go** of that body connection,…so you become free to **take** yourself somewhere pleasant your imagination chooses,…in order to **rest** your body's energy store,…refuelling, if you like,…**because** by doing this, right now,…**then** will encourage better sensations,…as *you* reduce the unwanted,…remove the unnecessary,…**reclaim** your sense of self,…as in doing so you straight away celebrate **clarity**,… a form of cleansing,…**with** fresh perspectives,…more **positive**,… fully connected to your deepest **strengths**,…**where** memories of your healthy body reside,…there you find pleasant **thoughts**,… accompanied by a sense of wellbeing,… **giv**ing so much vital **energy**,…which in turn creates an **increase in** positive thoughts,… and develops **healthier** physical changes,…for optimum sensations in each moment for your **sensory** appreciation,…because when you accept your willingness for positive **change**,…and for increased feelings of wellness,…**so** you notice how much better **you** feel,…**accept**ing how far you can travel using **your** mind,…to places of **joyfulness**,…where you find happiness,…**as well as** feel love,…of **acceptance** of all that is good for you,……..

so that now,…in your mind's eye,…realise the immense ability **you** have,…in your inner vision,…to see the most wonderful,…most beautiful images which **are** imaginable,…so what ever you see right now,…see it in colour,…be **calm**,…in detail,…in all it's beauty,…**embrace** the delight that accompanies the sights,…as you enjoy the pleasures of **these** visual **tranquilities**,…seeing shapes,…of light,…of shade,…with textures,…then perhaps an object as simple as a leaf,…or as complex as a leaf,…or even some scene so intricate and complex,…**you** wish to stare at it for a long time,….you **can** soak up the tiniest details,…maybe you're enthralled by the massive number of shades of each colour you see,…you can **cope** with seeing infinite shades and colours,…and **with** whatever you decide to **focus** on,…you're appreciating **on** a wise, deep level at the core of who you are, …how all that is **good** in this world,…for example,…right at this moment,…as you enjoy the **feelings** of sinking into a deeper, more comfortable relaxed state **of** calm,…with continuous **harmony** alongside longed for transformation,…just how you can imagine an almost incredible scene of nature,…say, **in** a rich and lush forest,…where ancient trees have stood silent and majestic for centuries,…**providing** shelter and nourishment for animals,…birds,…insects even the smallest creatures and organisms,… they are all part of a **healthy** system within the forest,…that keeps everything in tune and **living** well,…so should there be any unwanted elements **as** attempting to enter or cause trouble,…this complex forest system becomes *active*,…it uses the individual power of each thriving living thing,…and the combined synergic super *power* of all elements,… *removing* the *unwanted*,…the toxic,…to remove the unnecessary, …doing this *from* the very foundations of its wholeness,…just as in the same way, you can do this in *your whole self*,…..

all the while,…in your mind's eye,…you're walking through this vibrant, verdant forest,…noticing the different shades of greens and browns,…taking in the aromas of bark,… of moss,…combined with the enjoyable smells of healthy humid dampness,…blending with luscious smells of wood,…and ferns,…fresh humidity in the air,… *accept*ing without reservation,…*the* almost magical *ability* of all this,…*to* continue and *sustain* forest life,…whatever twists and turns occur within the *many* seasons and cycles of living,…during which all this time,…as you walk *deeper* into this marvellous tranquility,… so you feel safer,…and safe in the comfort of *realisations*,…this is your forest,…where you can do or be whatever you wish,…*for* as long as you wish,…because with each step you take along the forest path,…you fall *deeper* and deeper into a trance of *serenity*,… alongside true awe *and* wonder at the miraculous elements,…of *tremendous* continuation of forest life,…just as within your self you too are the same,…so much beauty,…with *love*,…with so much *of* all that is needed,…to maintain and build on *all that is good*,… banishing all that isn't,…without you having to do anything other than rest,…relax,…and *allow* this to happen,…furthermore,…as you let *this* happen right *now*,…as you walk through the forest,…*one* step after another,…taking deep, clear, constant breaths in,…in which you can savour the wood filled scents,…as they help clean your lungs,… whilst *energising* your whole self,…all the while *you're* enjoying time spent in such *agreeable* surroundings,……

thereafter the sun begins to shine **brighter** as you continue on **your** forest walk,…whereby you're **feeling** more warmth on your skin,…throughout your body,…blending into your body,…thoroughly warming,…genuinely caring,…changing the temperature of your whole self for the **better,**…so you **feel** better,…simply by letting it happen,…realising **you** can do that,…whilst continuing to relax,…as much as you **can**,…as well as visualising the forest walk,… and all the good **relax**ing sensations you feel **as** you continue,…because you can bask in the gentle soft warmth all around **you**,…comforting you,…caressing your body,…helping you to **feel** more calm,…with a deeper sense of well being,…a certainty in having a **tremendous** ability to remain still,… which is sometimes called **fortitude**,…providing resolute determination to have all good thoughts and feelings,…which for now,…as you continue to rest and relax,…you can allow yourself to drift into a deep healing sleep,…where you may dream of the forest,…of your courage,…resilience,…or you can choose to slowly and gently come back to full waking consciousness,…whilst your subconscious mind has made the positive changes within your self for the better,…creating feelings of invigoration,….you're more energised,…so much better able to manage,…as you're stronger,…much more determined,…happier…

> At this point end the induction by bringing the client back to consciousness or allowing them to continue into sleep proper. If you prefer you can use the standard awakening script near the beginning of the book.

Finding meaning in life

Use standard relaxation induction number 1.

Sometimes, as you move through life,…days add up to weeks,… weeks become months,…which turn into years,…then decades, ….when we arrive a time in our life where we consider what has happened with those years,……then we ask, what are we doing right now,….what for,….where am I going,……because it is good to ask these questions,…it's a healthy approach to making sure **you** are getting the most from life whilst planning the best future for yourself, …you **notice** you become healthier,…and perhaps **in** being decisive, …those you love notice in **subtle** ways,…you're happier **and** happier in yourself,…a **powerful** sense of yourself is emerging,…in **ways** that are good,…then for those people **that** matter to **you**,…they **are** finding you're **changing** for the better,…as you pass along each and every day,…**for** you're giving your attention to all that is **good**, that is beautiful, magical,…**finding** the changes inexplicable and yet marvellous,…**real**, in the very best ways we can experience **and** live, …so that we can feel the **deep** value in all the tremendous astonishingly awe inspiring **meaning**ful wonders given out **to** you as **your life** on this planet right now,…and yet,…and yet there are times when we yearn to connect with the good and the best things in life,… but instead, in the past, **this** has not always been how we are,… we've found a lack of **will**,…maybe the sparkle disappeared or didn't **happen**,…well, **now** the electric power of pleasure is in our grasp,… **and** we no longer feel alone,…you're moving **into the future** where you're much better position **for you** emotionally,…as **you** start to

feel as if you need to rekindle the buzz of excitement in spending time with activities, and with people, that **increasingly** lifts your sense of joy,…**happier**,…giving you the desired sense of purpose **and** ability to hold on to your reasons for being,…for **more** energy that puts the metaphorical fire in you to leap out of bed each morning,…yet **contented**,…so you can reconnect with those things you love that drive you **every** day,… to fulfil the promises you made yourself,…to be engaged with each **moment**,…to flourish as you endeavour to complete those chosen activities you enjoy within **the** range of what you are capable of,…so you can succeed now and in the **future** in those chosen tasks,…then your hopeful self **feels** a warm pride of success in your achievement,…**exciting**,…before you ponder on the future and how you will find new ways of finding your meaning **and** deciding your **enjoyable**, do-able tasks,…whatever they are,…whether they are for yourself only,…or whether they involve other likeminded good people,…or even whether they take you on a new adventurous journey wherein you meet new people,… experience new learnings,…you can **allow** good things to happen,… imagine **those ideas** right now,…because it is good **to** do that,…as we first must use our imagination **be**fore we embark on a **real** new way of being,…just as we can imagine, for example, feeling confident standing on a stage in front of many many people,… **because** giving a talk about an important subject that could improve the lives of many,…**your** mood will improve,…watching the faces of people in the audience listing to us with gratitude,…as your **subconscious mind** allows this to happen,…or just as you **will** imagine how to **make** an arduous sailing route on the ocean and hearing the cheers of well wishers on **these** shore as we sail home, …yes, your imagination is tremendously **important** in the choices and **changes** you make for yourself,…**in** every way,…as **your**

imagination propels you into a meaningful future which you have designed and which gives **character** and purpose and value to all you do,…improving your **personality**,…because what we choose to do matters to us,…**and** makes a difference to our feelings,…changing them into sturdy and solid **actions**, that give us fulfilment with the purest sense of joy, balance and well being,……

So right now, your subconscious mind can ask you to think consciously,…what are the factors that stir **you**,…those elements of your lived life which resonate with you,…maybe something you can **feel** good about,…perhaps something that creates **so much** happiness within yourself,…giving you a feel for what can be **better**, …or even something you have always dreamt of but up until **now** you have not followed that through,…now is the chance **you have** to make a difference in so many ways,…you can make a difference to yourself for the better,…a **rediscovered** part of you,…just as you can make a positive difference to the lives of others,…simply by **your** good and positive actions,…what ever they are,…you will feel a **sense** of delight deep down in knowing you have been the one person to have effected that goodness **of** change for the better,…in your heart,…in your head,…in your **purpose**,…in your whole being, …and you will feel the sense of meaning increasing in your life,…in your world,…the longer you follow that direction,…just as others will most likely notice how you have transformed situations and people, …as well as yourself,…because it's as if happiness is infectious, in a good way,…so your happiness spreads to those close to you,…as it follows that the atmosphere is lighter, more cheerful,…altogether better,……

Imagine, right now, one day of many for **your**self, where you wake up naturally then you want to get up as soon as possible,…fling yourself out of bed to begin the **tasks** you've set yourself,…whatever they **are**, they stimulate you and are **meaningful** to you,…imagine this,…**watch yourself being** engrossed in some activity or activities which cause you to feel so **happy**,…so involved,…you are happy to spend time doing these things,…imagine **your** whole day being filled with such delightful and engaging **activities**,…see yourself in your mind's eye doing these things,…**all day**,…with breaks for rest and sustenance,…your demeanour **brings** contentment,…fulfilment,…**purpose**,…I wonder what you've chosen to become engaged in,…it's absolutely fine whatever it is,…**because** we can all always change our minds and choose other things at some point,…that is a marvellous ability **you** have,…to change our minds,…and **do** something different if we **feel happier** doing so,……

as, I am sure **you** can take your time to **decide** exactly how you will change **your daily** routine,…in terms of how you will introduce new, **welcome changes** for yourself,…and maybe for others,…just as I'm sure these changes are going to make you happier,…**especially** in realising you can always keep on making **choices** whenever you decide the time is right to do so,…because whatever you choose that is **meaningful** to you,…so you will radiate pleasure internally **and** outwardly,……

Just allow your subconscious mind to spend some extra time during today dwelling on this words and statements, accepting the truth within them,…then forming a new plan,…a **remarkable** new plan,…that you can begin at once,….from now on,…

> At this point end the induction by bringing the client back to consciousness or allowing them to continue into sleep proper. If you prefer you can use the standard awakening script near the beginning of the book.

Creating resilience

Begin first by using standard relaxations 2, 3 or 4.

So lets begin with a physical relaxation,…allowing your muscles to soften,…feeling warm and comfortable,…finding a safe place where you will not be disturbed for around thirty minutes,…and ensuring your clothing is loose and comfortable,…**you** can now allow yourself to drift into a physical state of well being,…where you **are** beginning to let go of unwanted physical tensions,…being **resilient** whilst simply noticing places within **your** body,…where you may feel **inner** movement,…or tightness,…accepting these sensations as a form of **strength**,…which is malleable and **has** suppleness,…then allow your mind to move on to **more** parts of your body where you continue that relaxation,…using gentle inner **power,** and still breathing naturally and steadily,…breathing in and breathing out,…in and out,…just as you do **every day**, all day,…noticing your breath, …its rhythm, and length of the breath,…as those breaths encourage softening and relaxation within your muscles,…and in the whole of your body,…so **you** can feel yourself sinking deeper and deeper into that relaxation,…into a wonderful state,…deeper and then **make** that,…deeper,…peace, calm and harmony,…where your body rebalances encouraging wellness, **the** recovery of self,… rejuvenation of every single cell within your body,…bringing **wisest** optimism,…with increased energy,…all the while,…remaining steady and calm,…so as you listen to the sound of my voice, the sound of my voice helps you make **decisions** when to rest and relax,…like right now,…whilst your conscious mind can choose **to** listen to the sound of my voice,...as my voice is a **help**,...or your conscious mind can choose not to listen to the sound of my voice,...that's absolutely fine for **yourself**,...because your subconscious mind will listen to the voice pace, the tone, the rhythm, the style of speech, and **resolve** to choose all those helpful messages and suggestions the sound of my voice brings **to** you,...without you having to do anything at all other than stay pleasantly strong,...whilst you rest and relax,...so that the sound of my voice can be a background noise,...as your conscious thoughts drift and meander to other things,...whilst your subconscious mind processes the messages,...then decides and chooses,...and begins to take action for you,...so that **from now**, you can change your thoughts,...your feelings,...**you** behave for a better outcome,...in subtle, discreet ways,...or you **are** perhaps more obvious about it, or even both,...whatever your subconscious mind chooses, all is well,...as you are **more** sure of yourself, feeling immoveable and **tough**,...and if you can imagine in your mind's eye a packet of seeds from a gardening shop,...**sorting** through seeds of flowers, flowers that have never grown before,...yet have **life's** energy within them,...the picture on the front suggests your **tasks** will be enjoyable,...because the packet of seeds promise colourful flowers, strong and healthy, **with vibrant** petals,...petals of lush thickness,...and the messages on the packet talk of the **ease** of creating fragrances, and scents, and wildlife, and attraction of bees and honey,...**you** can imagine right now, as if you **are** planting these seeds in soil,...being **flexible, and** so you may visualise putting the seeds in plant pots,...or planting in the **hard** earth,...into the ground in a garden or a park,...over time,...with the nutrients of the soil,... water and sunlight, the seeds begin to grow roots,...deeper and deeper down into the earth,...as also,...a stem sprouts upwards,...a green stem appears above the ground,...and sometime later this stem is quite large and there are leaves,…then buds appear,… several buds,…and all the seeds **you** have planted **are** about to flower,…and I wonder if you are **able** to see that now as you visualise these flowers,…**to reflect** on how delicate and sensitive these seeds are,…**and** yet from these seeds have grown the most beautiful flowers that are now **blossom**ing,…can you see that **now**, …flowers of all colours, styles, shapes, sizes, and imagine the fragrances, the scents from these flowers,… **notice how** they are still so delicate,…**your** planting has helped create plants that are **powerful and strong**,…so perfect each and every one,…exactly the way they were meant to be when they were just tiny seeds,… **becoming** flowering plants,…and these flowers sway in the wind,… the hot summer wind,…sometimes quite gentle,…other times blowing a little **stronger**,…their stems allow the flowers to bend **with** graceful movements,…this way and that way to accommodate the force,…each and **everyday**,…and imagine now the rain is heavy,… heavier and heavier,…and notice how the flowers are **being** perfectly **resolute**,…turning their petals away from the direction of the rain and the wind,…and bend to allow themselves to stay **strong**,…and alive,…**providing** beauty,…and health to wildlife,… and later in the year **you** can visualise hail and snow,…falling upon the stems which are now **with**out their flowers,…and yet still full of **life**, and strong, resting over the cold period,…**to** bloom again the next year,…so in winter, whilst the temperatures **stay** low and cold, …and the ice and frost freeze the ground, still the inner seed,…lives on **determined**,…**powerful** in its silent strength,…then **when** the thaw comes,…so **you** can observe, the flowers springing to life once more,…they **need** to grow,…so they recover,…showing **resilience**, …grit,…absolute **determination** to continue,…despite adversity,… **and** just as the flower bends and turns away from the force which is unwanted,…as do trees bushes all living things,…so too **you can do this**,…with your inner resolutions and determination to keep yourself safe and strong,…realising at times it is far wiser to bend, even to hide,…and move away from sources of unwanted energies,…and in doing so,…**you** are becoming stronger,…showing firmness of spirit, …and nature,…and **know**ing this is the right thing to do,…the determination, **endurance**, reassurance, **is** all good for you,…you are doing the **right** things,…**and** in doing so **you are** feeling better about yourself, and forming a future where you can decide,…what you are **prepared** to tolerate,…so just as you are convinced you are doing the right thing,…in bending and adapting,…meandering away from unwanted, unnecessary, harmful sources of power and energy so you feel your inner courage growing,…combining with pride you can **feel** in yourself,…in making those decisions,…and that is **good** for you,…**having** changed so much, whilst maintaining your **integrity** and true self,……

as in the same way,…if you imagine going for walk in the countryside, maybe with friends, family or alone,…feeling happier and at one with yourself,…enjoying the sights and sounds and smells of the country,…identifying trees and bushes, looking for fruits,…in the distance you can see far away hills,…marked out by flint walls,…or by bushes creating quaint, attractive picture postcard images for you of the countryside as you walk along the path,… ambling at your own pace,…spending time with yourself,… **reconnect**ing to your true identity and the self that you are when calm and at one **with yourself**,…and all that surrounds you,…over time, **as** the sun rises in the sky and morning turns to noon,…**you** can **feel** your body tiring,…and yet you continue,…**proud**,…walking one step after another,…taking sustenance, and water when required,…**and** you keep walking with **cheerful** ness,…**and** as the sun makes its slow descent after its noon time highest point in the sky, you can see without looking,...that the afternoon is moving on, ...and whilst you're feeling so much more tired,... **your determination**, resilience **and** the ability you have to find hidden **energy** within,...**spurs** you on to walk further towards the town in the distance,...you're so very tired when **you** see the lights from the town in the distance,...**as** the sun has gone down,...and the voice within **you** says well done,...you **keep going** regardless,...you knew you had more,...on reaching the town and welcome refreshments you're overwhelmed with happiness, **confirming** you did the right thing,...showing **your**self and others the very **strength and power** that belongs to you,...the iron grit you have,...**to manage** difficult situations,...common sense **choices** whether to bend and adapt ,... or rest,...because you know how strong you can be,...and what is right for your overall well being,... in the present time and into the future,...

So rest your body,...imagine a delightful bedroom housing a sumptuous bed awaiting you,...and when you're ready, simply switch off the light,...and allow yourself to fall into a deep, long, healing sleep,...a creative sleep,...just as you can switch off from unwanted negative input from situations, experiences and people within your life,...and sleep soundly as you feel so good about yourself,... realising you can make wise choices,...and the decisions you make for yourself will help your future,...where you will know how resilient you really are,... feeling so good about yourself....

> At this point end the induction by bringing the client back to consciousness or allowing them to continue into sleep proper. If you prefer you can use the standard awakening script near the beginning of the book.

Final note

My wish is that everyone will benefit from the words and suggestions within this book. If you follow the guidelines in the first few chapters, practice a little before trying it for real, I'm sure your efforts will be effective and helpful. If at any time you think the induction isn't the right one, or the person isn't comfortable with it, then simply stop talking through that one. You could instead try using one of the four simple relaxations at the beginning of the book which are designed to allow the listener to gradually become relaxed. They take around five to ten minutes to complete.

The information provided in this book is designed to provide helpful tips and suggestions on the subject discussed. This book is not meant to be used, nor should it be used, to diagnose or treat any medical condition. For diagnosis or treatment of any medical problem, consult your own doctor. The publisher and author are not responsible for any specific health or allergy needs that may require medical supervision, and are not liable for any damages or negative consequences from any treatment, action, application or preparation, to any person reading or following the information in this book. Any references are provided for informational purposes only and do not constitute endorsement of any websites or other sources. Reader should be aware that the websites listed in this book may change.

Copyright © 2019 by Eileen M B Palmer
All rights reserved. This book or any portion thereof may not be reproduced or used in any manner whatsoever without the express written permission of the publisher except for the use of brief quotations in a book review.